Tracheal Surgery

Editors

ERICH HECKER
FRANK DETTERBECK

THORACIC SURGERY CLINICS

www.thoracic.theclinics.com

Consulting Editor
M. BLAIR MARSHALL

February 2014 • Volume 24 • Number 1

ELSEVIER

1600 John F. Kennedy Boulevard • Suite 1800 • Philadelphia, Pennsylvania, 19103-2899

http://www.theclinics.com

THORACIC SURGERY CLINICS Volume 24, Number 1
February 2014 ISSN 1547-4127, ISBN-13: 978-0-323-26684-0

Editor: John Vassallo (j.vassallo@elsevier.com)
Developmental Editor: Stephanie Carter

Thoracic Surgery Clinics (ISSN 1547-4127) is published quarterly by Elsevier Inc., 360 Park Avenue South, New York, NY 10010-1710. Months of publication are February, May, August, and November. Business and editorial offices: 1600 John F. Kennedy Boulevard, Suite 1800, Philadelphia, PA 19103-2899. Periodicals postage paid at New York, NY, and additional mailing offices. Subscription prices are $350.00 per year (US individuals), $453.00 per year (US institutions), $165.00 per year (US Students), $435.00 per year (Canadian individuals), $585.00 per year (Canadian institutions), $225.00 per year (Canadian and foreign students), $465.00 per year (foreign individuals), and $585.00 per year (foreign institutions). Foreign air speed delivery is included in all Clinics' subscription prices. All prices are subject to change without notice. **POSTMASTER:** Send address changes to Thoracic Surgery Clinics, Elsevier Health Sciences Division, Subscription Customer Service, 3251 Riverport Lane, Maryland Heights, MO 63043. **Customer Service (orders, claims, online, change of address): Telephone: 1-800-654-2452 (U.S. and Canada); 314-447-8871 (outside U.S. and Canada). Fax: 314-447-8029. Email: journalscustomerservice-usa@elsevier.com (for print support); journalsonlinesupport-usa@elsevier.com (for online support).**

Reprints. For copies of 100 or more, of articles in this publication, please contact Commercial Rights Department, Elsevier Inc., 360 Park Avenue South, New York, NY 10010-1710. Tel: 212-633-3874; Fax: 212-633-3820; E-mail: reprints@elsevier.com.

Thoracic Surgery Clinics is covered in *MEDLINE/PubMed (Index Medicus), EMBASE/Excerpta Medica, Science Citation Index Expanded (SciSearch®), Journal Citation Reports/Science Edition,* and *Current Contents®/Clinical Medicine.*

Printed and bound by CPI Group (UK) Ltd, Croydon, CR0 4YY

Transferred to digital print 2012

Contributors

CONSULTING EDITOR

M. BLAIR MARSHALL, MD
Associate Professor of Surgery, Georgetown University School of Medicine; Chief, Division of Thoracic Surgery, Department of Surgery, Georgetown University Medical Center, Washington, DC

EDITORS

ERICH HECKER, MD, PhD, MBA, FCCP
Chairman, Department of Thoracic Surgery, Thoraxzentrum Ruhrgebiet, Academic Hospital University Duisburg-Essen, Herne, Germany

FRANK DETTERBECK, MD, FACS, FCCP
Professor, Surgery, Yale University, New Haven, Connecticut

AUTHORS

FRANK BECKERS, MD, PhD
Assistant Director, Department of Thoracic Surgery, Lung Clinic, Hospital of Cologne, University of Witten/Herdecke, Cologne, Germany

DIRK BEHRINGER, MD, PhD
Professor, Chief and Head, Department of Hematology, Oncology and Palliative Care, Thoraxzentrum Ruhrgebiet, Augusta Kliniken, Bochum, Germany

BEATE E.M. BRAND-SABERI, MD, PhD
Professor, Department of Anatomy and Molecular Embryology, Institute of Anatomy, Ruhr University Bochum, Bochum, Germany

KAID DARWICHE, MD, PhD
Assistant Director, Department of Interventional Pneumology, Ruhrlandklinik, University Hospital, University Duisburg-Essen, Essen, Germany

FRANK DETTERBECK, MD, FACS, FCCP
Professor, Surgery, Yale University, New Haven, Connecticut

LUTZ FREITAG, MD, PhD, FCCP
Professor of Pulmonary Medicine, Chief, Department of Interventional Pneumology, Ruhrlandklinik, University Hospital, University Duisburg-Essen, Essen, Germany

ERICH HECKER, MD, PhD, MBA, FCCP
Chairman, Department of Thoracic Surgery, Thoraxzentrum Ruhrgebiet, Academic Hospital University Duisburg-Essen, Herne, Germany

SASCHA C.A. HERBER, MD, PhD
Chief and Head, Department of Radiology, Catholic Clinics Koblenz-Montabaur, University Teaching Hospital, Koblenz, Germany

MARTIN HÜRTGEN, MD, PhD
Chief and Head, Department of Thoracic Surgery, Catholic Clinics Koblenz-Montabaur, University Teaching Hospital, Koblenz, Germany

ILHAN INCI, MD
Associate Professor, Department of Thoracic Surgery, University Hospital, University of Zurich, Zurich, Switzerland

PHILIPP JUNGEBLUTH, MD
Division of Ear, Nose, and Throat (CLINTEC), Advanced Center for Translational Regenerative Medicine (ACTREM), Karolinska Institutet, Stockholm, Sweden

KLAUS JUNKER, MD, PhD
Professor, Chief and Head, Institute of Pathology, Bremen Central Hospital, Bremen, Germany

STEFAN KÖNEMANN, MD, PhD
Chief and Head, Department of Radiotherapy, Thoraxzentrum Ruhrgebiet, Strahlentherapiezentrum Bochum, Bochum, Germany

ARIS KORYLLOS, MD
Thoracic Surgery, Lung Clinic, Hospital of Cologne, University of Witten/Herdecke, Cologne, Germany

CHRISTIAN KUGLER, MD, PhD
Chief and Head, Department of Thoracic Surgery, LungenClinic Großhansdorf, Großhansdorf, Germany

GUNDA LESCHBER, MD, PhD
Chief and Head, Department of Thoracic Surgery, ELK Berlin Chest Hospital, Berlin, Germany

CORINNA LUDWIG, MD, PhD
Assistant Director, Department of Thoracic Surgery, Lung Clinic, Hospital of Cologne, University of Witten/Herdecke, Cologne, Germany

PAOLO MACCHIARINI, MD, PhD
Professor, Division of Ear, Nose, and Throat (CLINTEC), Advanced Center for Translational Regenerative Medicine (ACTREM), Karolinska Institute, Stockholm, Sweden

CLEMENS MÄNNLE, MD, PhD
Assistant Director, Department of Anesthesiology and Intensive Care, Thoraxklinik, University Hospitals, Heidelberg, Germany

THORSTEN SCHÄFER, MD, PhD
Professor, Institute of Clinical Physiology, Institute of Physiology, Ruhr University Bochum, Bochum, Germany

FRANZ STANZEL, MD, PhD, FCCP
Chief and Head, Department of Pneumology, Lung Clinic Hemer, Hemer, Germany

ERICH STOELBEN, MD, PhD
Professor, Chief and Head, Deaprtment of Thoracic Surgery, Lung Clinic, Hospital of Cologne, University of Witten/Herdecke, Cologne, Germany

JAN VOLMERIG, MD, PhD, FEBTS, MBA
Assistant Director, Department of Thoracic Surgery, Thoraxzentrum Ruhrgebiet, Academic Hospital University Duisburg-Essen, Herne, Germany

WALTER WEDER, MD, PhD
Professor, Clinic Director, Department of Thoracic Surgery, University Hospital, University of Zurich, Zurich, Switzerland

STEFAN WELTER, MD, PhD
Department of Thoracic Surgery and Endoscopy, Ruhrlandklinik, University Clinic, University of Duisburg-Essen, Essen, Germany

KLAUS WIEDEMANN, MD, PhD
Retired, Formerly: Professor of Anesthesiology, Department of Anesthesiology and Intensive Care, Thoraxklinik, University Hospitals, Heidelberg, Germany

AHMAD ZEESHAN, MD
Section of Thoracic Surgery, Academic Hospital University Duisburg-Essen, Herne, Germany

Contents

Preface xi

Erich Hecker and Frank Detterbeck

Trachea: Anatomy and Physiology 1

Beate E.M. Brand-Saberi and Thorsten Schäfer

The windpipe (trachea) is a tube of 12 cm length connecting the larynx to the principal bronchi that lead to the lungs. The main functions of the trachea comprise air flow into the lungs, mucociliary clearance, and humidification and warming of air. Mucociliary clearance is achieved by kinocilia and goblet cells in the mucosa, and by tracheal glands. The trachea develops from the endodermal lining of the foregut in interaction with the visceral mesoderm. During adult life, different types of stem cells reside in the mucosal epithelium and glandular ducts. Recently, cholinergic chemosensory cells have been described in the trachea.

Pathology of Tracheal Tumors 7

Klaus Junker

Malignant involvement of the trachea predominantly results from direct spread of neighboring tumors to the tracheal wall. Primary tracheal malignancies show a low incidence of approximately 0.1 in every 100,000 persons per year, squamous cell carcinomas and adenoid cystic carcinomas accounting for about two-thirds of adult primary tracheal tumors. The etiology of squamous cell carcinoma and its premalignant lesions is strongly associated with tobacco smoking. Patients with tracheal malignancies show an unfavorable prognosis, with reported 5- and 10-year survival rates of 5% to 15% and 6% to 7%, respectively, for all types of tracheal carcinoma.

Anesthesia and Gas Exchange in Tracheal Surgery 13

Klaus Wiedemann and Clemens Männle

Tracheobronchial surgery constitutes a challenge to the anesthetist because it involves the anatomic structures dedicated to bulk gas transport. Common approaches to airway management and gas exchange for extrathoracic and intrathoracic airway surgery are reviewed, with due regard to less common methods thought crucial for specific procedures. Tracheal surgery, beyond sharing the airways, requires sharing with the surgeon ideas on preoperative assessment, on the impact on gas exchange of induction across compromised airways, and of emergence from anesthesia with airways altered by surgical repair. Mutual understanding is essential to prevent, rapidly identify, and correct imminent loss of airway viability.

Endoscopic Treatment of Tracheal Stenosis 27

Lutz Freitag and Kaid Darwiche

For all cases of tracheal obstructions, surgery should be considered first. Interventional endoscopic procedures can provide immediate relief. Intraluminally growing tumors can be resected with laser, argon-plasma coagulation, an electrosurgical knife or cryo-probe. Photodynamic therapy of smaller tracheal tumors can be curative. Narrowing from intramural tumor growth or wall destruction requires internal splinting with an airway stent. Scar strictures can be dilated with balloons, but the biotrauma may stimulate new scarring. In benign strictures and malacias, tracheal stents should only be placed if all other methods are exhausted. Complications including stent migration, mucostasis, halitosis, and granulation tissue development must be considered. Most important for a good outcome is a multidisciplinary approach.

Repair of Tracheobronchial Injuries **41**

Stefan Welter

Videos of complete intraluminal repair of a iatrogenic tracheal laceration and expiratory tracheal collapse in the region of a former tracheal membrane laceration accompany this article

Tracheobronchial injuries (TBIs) are caused by blunt, penetrating injury or by iatrogenic damage. Most injuries are life threatening and need early and skillful airway management. Bronchoscopy remains the gold standard of diagnosis. Penetrating TBI always needs blunt trauma, and iatrogenic TBI sometimes needs surgical exploration and reconstruction, which is performed after sparing debridement with primary repair and wound closure. Prognosis mainly depends on associated injuries and comorbidities in terms of tracheal membrane laceration.

Tracheomalacia **51**

Christian Kugler and Franz Stanzel

Tracheomalacia is excessive collapsibility of the trachea, typically during expiration. Congenital forms are associated with severe symptoms. Milder forms often present after the neonatal period. Adult malacia is mostly associated with chronic obstructive pulmonary disease. Functional bronchoscopy is still not standardized. Dynamic airway CT is a promising tool for noninvasive diagnosis. Bronchoscopy and stent insertion lead to significant improvement, but with a high complication rate. Surgical lateropexia, tracheal resection, and surgical external stabilization are options. Tracheoplasty seems to be the best choice for selected cases of adult malacia. The most commonly performed surgery in children is aortopexy.

Benign Stenosis of the Trachea **59**

Erich Stoelben, Aris Koryllos, Frank Beckers, and Corinna Ludwig

Benign stenosis of trachea results mainly from tracheotomy, ventilation, or trauma. The combination of a defect of the mucosa or the tracheal wall and infection produce secondary scar tissue healing with shrinkage of the tracheal lumen or instability of the tracheal wall. Standard of treatment consists of resection of the pathologic segment of the trachea with end-to-end anastomosis. In case of involvement of the larynx, partial resections of the anterior cricoid cartilage or division of the larynx with tracheolaryngeal silicone stents are used. Short-term and long-term results are satisfying considering some technical recommendations.

Laryngotracheal Resection and Reconstruction **67**

Ahmad Zeeshan, Frank Detterbeck, and Erich Hecker

Patients with tracheal stenosis can experience life-threatening dyspnea. When the stenosis is close to the larynx, management can be challenging. Non-definitive palliative measures should be kept to a minimum as they can make definitive management more complicated. Specialized techniques of resection and reconstruction of high tracheal lesions are available, and lead to excellent relief of symptoms. A detailed knowledge of the anatomy, the extent of the stenosis, and careful attention to surgical technique is crucial. Excellent results can be achieved in experienced centers that are able to anticipate and thus avoid complications that can be difficult to manage.

Treatment Approaches to Primary Tracheal Cancer 73

Dirk Behringer, Stefan Könemann, and Erich Hecker

A patient identified with tracheal cancer benefits most from evaluation by an experienced center and an extensive effort to assess the possibility of a complete surgical resection as the most efficient treatment option for cure. Localized, nonoperable disease may still be controlled by combined modality using chemotherapy and concurrent radiation.

Carinal Resection and Sleeve Pneumonectomy 77

Walter Weder and Ilhan Inci

Carinal resection and sleeve pneumonectomy are rare procedures and challenging issues in thoracic surgery. In spite of the knowledge of the technique, the incidence of postoperative complications is higher compared with standard resections. Adequate patient selection, improved anesthetic management and surgical technique, and better postoperative management might reduce the rate of postoperative morbidity and mortality.

Extended Tracheal Resections 85

Erich Hecker and Jan Volmerig

There is no universally valid definition of the extent of tracheal resections that would be considered “extended.” Underlying disease, necessary length of resection, anatomic localization, and chosen surgical approach account for a manifold interdependency. Existing data suggest a “cutoff margin” of 4 cm or more, referring to the likelihood of complications and necessity of additional mobilization maneuvers. This overview outlines worldwide experiences and the surgical variety of possibilities, as well as their execution and appropriate use.

Airway Transplantation 97

Philipp Jungebluth and Paolo Macchiarini

No definitive solution has been discovered for replacing long segments or the entire trachea in humans. Most of this challenge stems from the specific function and mechanics that are almost impossible to replicate except in the setting of an allotransplantation, which requires lifelong immunosuppressive medication. Recently, tissue engineering provided significant evidence concerning the next promising therapeutic alternative for tracheal replacement. Underlying mechanism and pathways of cell-surface interactions, cell migration, and differentiation are essential to understand the complexity of tracheal tissue regeneration. Tracheal replacement remains challenging but initial steps toward an ideal therapeutic concept have been made.

Management of Tracheal Surgery Complications 107

Gunda Leschber

Complications in tracheal surgery are not uncommon but generally do not influence the final result. Most patients benefit from tracheal resections and mortality is low.

Risk factors for complications are reoperations, preoperative tracheostomy, and lengthy resections. Precise information about the extent of the diseased tracheal part as well as thorough planning of the operative procedure, meticulous dissection, and knowledge of release maneuvers by an experienced thoracic surgeon will diminish the risk of adverse effects. Granuloma formation is the most common event observed postoperatively, whereas dehiscence and restenosis or the potentially fatal bleeding from a tracheo-innominate artery fistula occurs less frequently.

Treatment of Malignant Tracheoesophageal Fistula **117**

Martin Hürtgen and Sascha C.A. Herber

This article addresses the treatment of malignant enterorespiratory fistulas, especially malignant tracheoesophageal fistula (mTEF). mTEF typically occurs after radiochemotherapy for advanced esophageal cancer. Life expectancy is measured in months after successful treatment, and in days to weeks with a persistent fistula. To stop repeated episodes of aspiration and septic pneumonia, single or double stenting of the esophagus and trachea with self-expandable coated stents is the established palliative treatment. The indications, techniques, and pitfalls of esophageal and tracheal stenting are described. Surgical interventions are justified only in very select cases, so this article focuses on interventional rather than surgical treatment.

Index **129**

THORACIC SURGERY CLINICS

FORTHCOMING ISSUES

May 2014
Robotic Surgery
Bernard Park, MD, *Editor*

August 2014
Neuroendocrine Tumors of the Lung
Pier Luigi Filosso, MD, *Editor*

November 2014
Aggressive Surgical Therapy for Advanced Lung Cancer
Raja Flores, MD, *Editor*

RECENT ISSUES

November 2013
Evolving Therapies in Esophageal Carcinoma
Wayne L. Hoffstetter, MD, *Editor*

August 2013
Lung Cancer, Part II: Surgery and Adjuvant Therapies
Jean Deslauriers, MD, F. Griffith Pearson, MD, and Farid M. Shamji, MD, *Editors*

May 2013
Lung Cancer, Part I: Screening, Diagnosis, and Staging
Jean Deslauriers, MD, F. Griffith Pearson, MD, and Farid M. Shamji, MD, *Editors*

RELATED INTEREST

Surgical Clinics of North America, Volume 92, Issue 5 (October 2012)
Contemporary Management of Esophageal Malignancy
Chadrick E. Denlinger, MD, and Carolyn E. Reed, MD, *Editors*
Available at www.surgical.theclinics.com

Preface

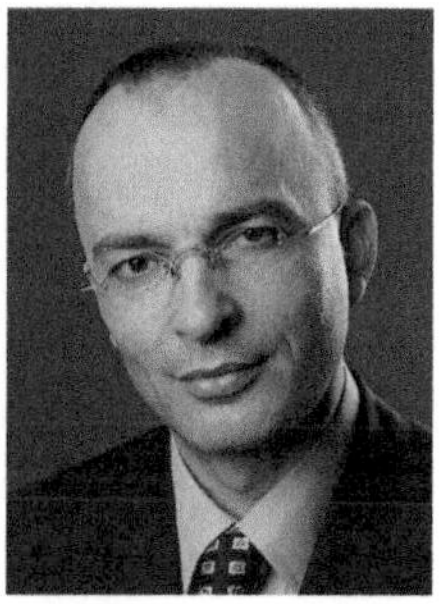

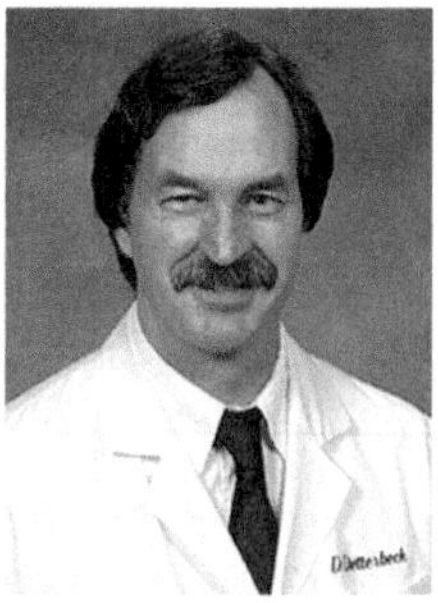

Erich Hecker, MD Frank Detterbeck, MD

Editors

The topic of tracheal surgery was last addressed by the *Thoracic Surgery Clinics* in 2003 (at that time called *Chest Surgery Clinics of North America*). That issue contained contributions from, and was dedicated to, Hermes C. Grillo, in recognition of his major contributions to the development of modern tracheal surgery. The field has advanced significantly since then, now without Dr Grillo, but his impact is no less prominent today.

This current issue is the result of a recent Symposium on Tracheal Surgery (Herne, Germany in 2011), which was organized to mark the intersection of three related anniversaries: 130 years since the first tracheal resection,[1] 100 years since the first resection of a tracheal cancer,[2] and 30 years since the establishment of the Thoracic Surgery Center in the Ruhr region of Germany.[3] This Symposium involved an up-to-date review of the literature and insights gained from the personal experience of the invited experts in each area of tracheal surgery.

The goal of this issue is to present a compilation of the available evidence and experience in tracheal surgery that should guide our decision-making and management of patients with tracheal conditions. We hope that this review is helpful, because the incidence of surgical interventions for tracheal problems remains relatively rare at 0.2 per 100,000 inhabitants, despite the fact that the first tracheotomy was published 3500 years ago.

We thank the publisher for making it possible to publish this comprehensive review of the state of the art of the anatomy, physiology, pathology, anesthetic management, surgical and nonsurgical interventions, including advances in tissue engineering related to the management of tracheal conditions.

Erich Hecker, MD
Department of Thoracic Surgery
Thoraxzentrum Ruhrgebiet
Herne, Germany

Frank Detterbeck, MD
Yale University
New Haven, CT, USA

E-mail addresses:
e.hecker@evk-herne.de (E. Hecker)
frank.detterbeck@yale.edu (F. Detterbeck)

REFERENCES

1. Gluck T. Die prophylaktische Resektion der Trachea. Arch Klin Chir 1881;26:427–36.
2. Soerensen J. Zwei Fälle von Totalexstirpation der Trachea wegen Karzinom. Arch Laryngol Rhinol 1915;29:188–204.
3. Tracheachirurgie–Festaktsymposium 2011. Klinik für Thoraxchirurgie, Thoraxzentrum Ruhrgebiet; 2011.

Thorac Surg Clin 24 (2014) xi
http://dx.doi.org/10.1016/j.thorsurg.2013.10.007
1547-4127/14/$ – see front matter

Trachea: Anatomy and Physiology

Beate E.M. Brand-Saberi[a,*], Thorsten Schäfer[b]

KEYWORDS

• Macroscopic and microscopic anatomy • Morphogenesis • Tracheal stem cells • Physiology • Function

KEY POINTS

- The trachea is a tube made up of cartilage, connective tissue, smooth muscle, and a mucosal layer connecting the larynx to the principal bronchi and finally to the lungs.
- The tracheal mucosa consists of a pseudostratified columnar epithelium with kinocilia and goblet cells, supported by a lamina propria containing tracheal glands.
- Morphogenesis of the trachea depends on epithelial-mesenchymal interactions of the endodermal trachea and the mesoderm-derived mesenchyme surrounding it.
- The mucosal epithelium and the ducts of the tracheal glands contain different types of stem cells.
- The main functions of the trachea comprise air flow into the lungs, mucociliary clearance, and humidification and warming of the air.

ANATOMIC OVERVIEW OF THE TRACHEA

The trachea (windpipe) is a semiflexible tube of 1.5 to 2 cm in width and 10 to 13 cm in length, reaching from the lower portion of the larynx approximately at the level of the sixth to seventh cervical vertebra to the fourth to fifth thoracic vertebra, where it bifurcates to form the two bronchi for the lungs. The tracheal wall consists of up to 20 incomplete rings of hyaline cartilage forming the anterior and lateral circumference, and smooth muscle at the posterior side, which are both embedded into a fibrous membrane of elastic connective tissue (**Fig. 1**). The muscle contains transverse and longitudinal fibers; the transverse fibers connect the ends of the cartilaginous rings posteriorly and are termed m. trachealis. Seromucinous tracheal glands are located in the connective tissue between the epithelial layer and the cartilage, sometimes also on the outer side, and are found abundantly exterior to the tracheal muscle. The function of the glands that open via ducts on the inner surface of the trachea is to lubricate the inner lining of the trachea. The epithelium consists of a pseudostratified columnar epithelium with kinocilia and goblet cells that also produce a mucous film (**Fig. 2**). The direction of the beat of the kinocilia toward the larynx results in the transport of particulates and cell detritus away from the lungs and its elimination from the body.

MORPHOGENESIS OF THE TRACHEA

During the fourth week of development, the trachea develops initially from the ventral foregut epithelium forming the tracheobronchial diverticulum, and grows caudally before branching into the lung buds that will later elongate to form the principal bronchi. The inner lining of the trachea is thus of endodermal origin. However, it is an excellent example of epithelial-mesenchymal interactions that occur commonly during organogenesis, because the endodermal tube undergoes morphogenetic movements such as growth and branching

The authors have nothing to disclose.

[a] Department of Anatomy and Molecular Embryology, Institute of Anatomy, Ruhr University Bochum, Universitaetsstrasse 150, Bochum 44801, Germany; [b] Helios Klinik Hagen-Ambrock, Institute of Clinical Physiology, Institute of Physiology, Ruhr University Bochum, Universitaetsstrasse 150, Bochum 44801, Germany
* Corresponding author.
E-mail address: beate.brand-saberi@rub.de

Thorac Surg Clin 24 (2014) 1–5
http://dx.doi.org/10.1016/j.thorsurg.2013.09.004

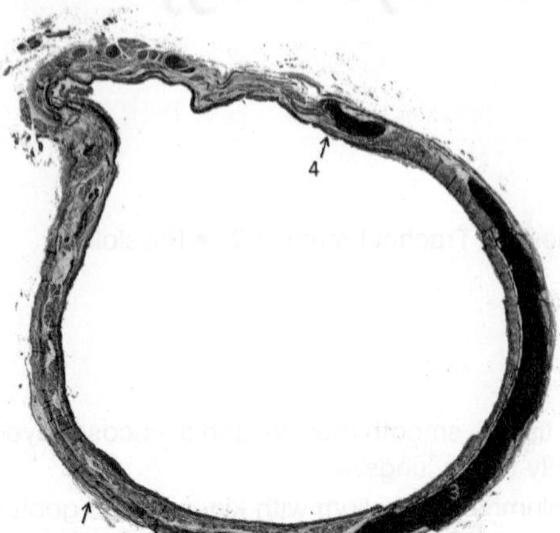

Fig. 1. Transverse section of a human trachea with fibromuscular portion (paries membranaceus; 1) and tracheal cartilage (3); the seromucinous tracheal glands (2) are located in the connective tissue subjacent to the inner lining. The tunica mucosa (4) consists of the pseudostratified columnar epithelium shown in **Fig. 2**, and the lamina propria. The tunica adventitia is labeled as 5. (Azan staining, original magnification × 40).

only under the influence of the surrounding splanchnic mesoderm (**Fig. 3**). The interactions are based on signals from the major signaling pathways such as fibroblast growth factor 10, Sprouty, epidermal growth factor, insulin-like growth factor, hepatocyte growth factor, and transcription factors.[1] During the fourth week of development, the trachea branches to form the right and the left lung bud. The development of the trachea thus forms the prerequisite for the formation of the lungs by repeated rounds of bifurcation events (**Fig. 4**).

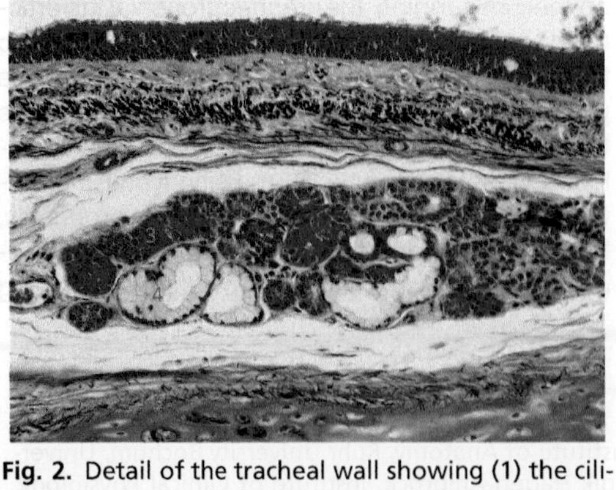

Fig. 2. Detail of the tracheal wall showing (1) the ciliated pseudostratified columnar epithelium, (2) elastic fibers of the lamina propria, tracheal glands with serous (3) and mucinous (4) acini, and (5) hyaline tracheal cartilage. (Goldner staining, original magnification × 200).

RECENT HISTOLOGIC FINDINGS

A detailed analysis of the pseudostratified mucosal epithelium of the trachea has revealed the presence of several highly specialized and less well-defined cell types. The most common distinction is made between the "brush cells" and the neuroendocrine cells resembling the enteroendocrine cells of the gastrointestinal tract, neuroendocrine cells being dispersed in the respiratory epithelium. The function of the neuroendocrine cells in the respiratory tract is currently under debate; mechanosensitive functions and O_2-sensing functions[2] have been suggested. In contrast to the enteroendocrine cells, the chemosensory function of the neuroendocrine cells in the respiratory tract has not yet been proved. The non-neuroendocrine cells of the respiratory tract have been termed brush cells, and are solitary chemosensory cells in the upper airways. Surprisingly, cells expressing the molecular components of the taste transduction pathway display the ultrastructural morphology of the brush cells.[3] The term brush cell reflects the presence of apical microvilli containing villin and fimbrin.[4] Recently, cholinergic chemosensory cells have been described in the trachea[5–7] by expression of relevant receptors and components of the bitter taste transduction pathway. These cells are connected to afferent fibers of the vagal nerve via nicotinic acetylcholine receptors. These cholinergic brush cells were demonstrated to affect the control of breathing,[5] and are thus functional in safeguarding the lower airways by sensing the composition of the luminal fluid inside the trachea and the bronchi.

TRACHEAL STEM CELLS

As the epithelium of the airways is exposed to the environment with the risk of injury, it must be able to physiologically regenerate. During this process, a subpopulation of the basal cells in the pseudostratified columnar epithelium is activated, and replaces the sloughed or injured surface cells.[8–10] The stem/progenitor cells can be characterized by the presence of transcription factor Trp-63 (p63) and cytokeratins 5 and 14.[11] Trp-63 is involved in the development of the respiratory and other epithelia, in particular the establishment of the basal cells.[12] In contrast to rodents in which these stem/progenitor cells are only present in the trachea, in humans they occur throughout the respiratory tract, including the small bronchi. Basal cells can develop into ciliated surface cells and Clara cells which, as Clara cells give rise to goblet cells, can be considered multipotent.

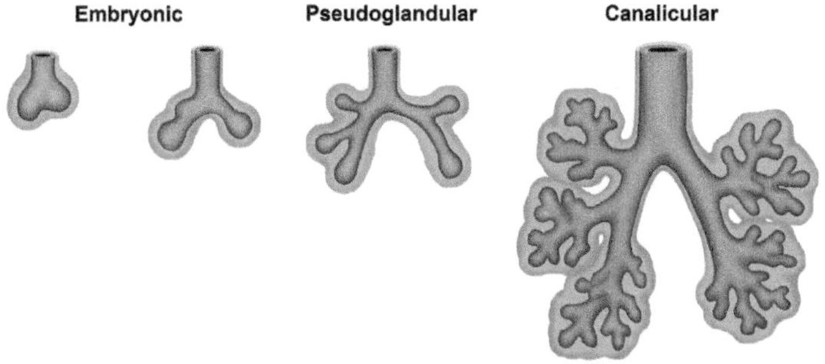

Fig. 3. Ventral view of embryonic trachea and lung development. The endodermal lining of the tracheobronchial diverticulum is depicted in light brown and the splanchnic mesoderm surrounding it is depicted in gray. Growth and bifurcations occur in a sequence of epithelial-mesenchymal interactions involving signaling molecules and transcription factors. Lung development thus depends on the formation of the tracheobronchial bud, and occurs in several phases (embryonic, pseudoglandular, canalicular). (*Courtesy of* Helga Schulze, Bochum, Germany.)

Despite early reports and a long history during which stem/progenitor cells had already been described in the seromucinous glands lining the airways,[13,14] more recently a new type of stem/progenitor cell has been described in the trachea of the mouse,[15] which is localized in the ducts of the tracheal glands. The gland duct cells have been isolated and shown to be multipotent stem/progenitor cell populations for the murine airway epithelium that can give rise to serous and mucous tubules, duct cells, and ciliated surface epithelium. What makes them unique is their capability to survive severe hypoxic-ischemic injury. Although the situation differs between mouse and humans,[14,16] these findings contribute important insights into the physiology of the tracheal epithelium, in particular in the pathologic setting.

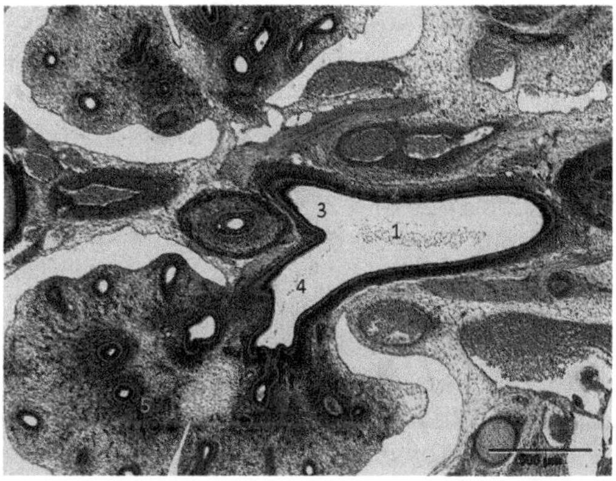

Fig. 4. Frontal section of a human embryo of 22.5 mm (Carnegie stage 21). The trachea (1) with cartilage blastemas (2) has divided into the right (3) and the left (4) principal bronchus. (5) indicates the developing left lung, and (6) the developing right lung. (Hematoxylin-eosin staining, original magnification × 40). (*Courtesy of* Professor Dr Klaus Hinrichsen, Bochum, Germany.)

PHYSIOLOGIC OVERVIEW OF THE TRACHEA

The trachea

- Conducts air between the larynx and the bronchi
- Exchanges heat and moisture
- Removes particles

AIR TRANSPORT IN THE TRACHEA

The transport of air is critically dependent on the inner diameter of the trachea. The resistance to flow through a tube, represented by the law of Hagen-Poiseuille, is inversely proportional to the radius of the tube raised to the fourth power, as long as the flow is laminar. At higher flow rates the flow may become turbulent, which further increases the resistance (**Fig. 5**). Mucosal swelling, constriction of airway muscles, or tumors that reduce the airway space, but also endotracheal tubes, considerably increase the resistance to airflow: a 50% reduction of the inner diameter increases the resistance 16-fold, and during turbulent flow up to 32-fold.[17]

AIR CONDITIONING

During inspiration the upper airways warm and humidify the inspired air. This process is very efficient. During quiet breathing at room temperature, air is completely warmed up to 37°C and humidified to 100% saturation shortly distal of the bifurcation; this is called the isothermal saturation point. The drier and colder the inspired air is, the more this point moves to the lung periphery, inducing dehydration and cooling of the lung tissue.[18] Extreme mountaineering or mountain biking, for example, combines inspiration of cold and dry air with high levels of minute ventilation, leading to stress on the lung tissue. In addition,

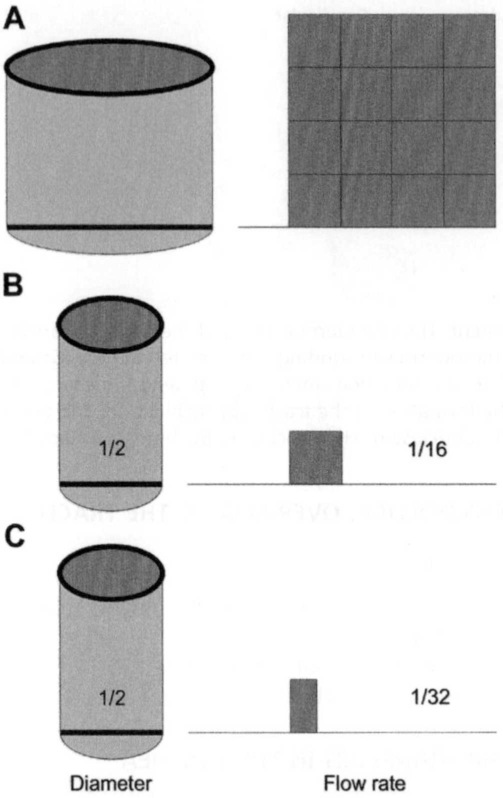

Fig. 5. Effect of reduction of the tube diameter on the flow rate (at constant pressures) according to the law of Hagen-Poiseuille. Halving of the diameter of a tube (*A*) reduces the flow rate to 1/16 under the conditions of laminar flow (*B*) and to 1/32 during turbulent flow (*C*).

however, bypassing the upper airways with a tracheostomy or endotracheal tubes may lead to cooling and drying of lung tissue, unless the inspired air is warmed and humidified.[17]

Room air at a temperature of 22°C and 50% relative humidity approximately contains 10 mg/L H_2O and will have absorbed an additional 34 mg/L at the isothermal saturation point. Expired air cools down to approximately 32°C at the nostrils and still contains 34 mg/L moisture at 100% relative humidity. This amount causes a daily water loss of at least 240 mL as part of the "perspiratio insensibilis," the unnoticed loss of fluid via the skin and the lungs. The energy requirement to compensate for evaporative cooling equals approximately 600 kJ per day, which is about 10% of the total heat production of the body.[19]

REMOVAL OF INSPIRED DEBRIS AND ASPIRATED MICROORGANISMS

Tracheobronchial glands produce a mucin-rich secretion that forms a protective barrier between the epithelium and the environment. This secretion is largely controlled by the autonomic nervous system, modulated by numerous inflammatory mediators.[20] These mediators form 2, possibly 3, layers: a sol layer is next to the epithelium, making ciliary beating possible. The sol layer is covered by the mucus or gel layer, possibly separated by a layer of surfactant. The mucus collects debris and microorganisms, and is transported orally by the mechanical forces of coordinated ciliary beating and the airflow during expiration. Mucus production and mucociliary transport capacity are higher in the small airways than in the central airways, where transport by expiratory airflow is higher.[21] This airflow transport mainly depends on the airflow velocity during expiration, determined by the airway diameter and the difference between intrapulmonary and ambient pressure. The mucus viscosity varies depending on shear forces, and may decrease by a factor of up to 500 during coughing, which is explained by a realignment of macromolecules by the applied force.[21]

Nishino and colleagues[22] found at least 6 different responses to stimulation of tracheal mucosa by injection of distilled water, examined under different levels of enflurane anesthesia:

- Cough reflex (most sensitive)
- Apneic reflex (most resistant to deepening anesthesia)
- Expiration reflex
- Spasmodic, panting breathing
- Slowing of breathing
- Rapid shallow breathing

A cough begins with a closure of the glottis, followed by an isometric contraction of the expiratory muscles, which generates a high intrathoracic pressure. Sudden opening of the glottis creates a burst of expiratory airflow, transporting mucus orally. Huffs have a similar effect on mucus transport. Huffs start with a fast, dynamic expiration. The glottis remains open throughout the maneuver.[21]

In conclusion, the functions of the trachea by far exceed the simple conduction of air between the larynx and the lungs: The trachea plays an important role in the protection of the sensitive lung tissue from injuries and invasion by microorganisms. Pathologic or iatrogenic restrictions of the tracheal lumen severely increase the airway resistance and, thus, the patient's work of breathing.

ACKNOWLEDGMENTS

The authors wish to thank Annegrit Schlichting and Asta Schiffgen for excellent technical support,

Helga Schulze for art work, and Abdulatif Al Haj, M.Sc., for photographs of histologic sections.

REFERENCES

1. Warburton D, Schwarz M, Tefft D, et al. The molecular basis of lung morphogenesis. Mech Dev 2000; 92:55–81.
2. Cutz E, Yeger H, Pan J. Pulmonary neuroendocrine cell system in pediatric lung disease—recent advances. Pediatr Dev Pathol 2007;10(6):419–35.
3. Merigo F, Benati D, Tizziano M, et al. α-Gustducin immunoreactivity in the airways. Cell Tissue Res 2005;319(2):211–9.
4. Höfer D, Drenckhahn D. Identification of brush cells in the alimentary and respiratory system by antibodies to villin and fimbrin. Histochemistry 1992; 98(4):237–42.
5. Kummer W, Lips KS, Pfeil U. The epithelial cholinergic system of the airways. Histochem Cell Biol 2008;130(2):219–34.
6. Krasteva G, Canning BJ, Hartmann P, et al. Cholinergic chemosensory cells in the trachea regulate breathing. Proc Natl Acad Sci U S A 2011;108(23): 9478–83.
7. Krasteva G, Kummer W. "Tasting" the airway lining fluid. Histochem Cell Biol 2012;138:365–83.
8. Schoch KG, Lori A, Burns KA, et al. A subset of mouse tracheal epithelial basal cells generates large colonies in vitro. Am J Physiol Lung Cell Mol Physiol 2004;286:L631–42.
9. Hong KU, Reynolds SD, Watkins S, et al. Basal cells are a multipotent progenitor capable of renewing the bronchial epithelium. Am J Pathol 2004;164:577–88.
10. Hong KU, Reynolds SD, Watkins S, et al. In vivo differentiation potential of tracheal basal cells: evidence for multipotent and unipotent subpopulations. Am J Physiol Lung Cell Mol Physiol 2004; 286:L643–9.
11. Rock JR, Onaitis MW, Rawlins EL, et al. Basal cells as stem cells of the mouse trachea and human airway epithelium. Proc Natl Acad Sci U S A 2009; 106:12771–5.
12. Daniely Y, Liao G, Dixon D, et al. Critical role of p63 in the development of a normal esophageal and tracheobronchial epithelium. Am J Physiol Cell Physiol 2004;287:C171–81.
13. Engelhart JF, Schlossberg H, Yankaskas JR, et al. Progenitor cells of the adult human airway involved in submucosal gland development. Development 1995;121:2031–46.
14. Liu XM, Engelhardt JF. The glandular stem/progenitor cell niche in airway development and repair. Proc Am Thorac Soc 2008;5:682–8.
15. Hegab A, Ha VL, Gilbert JL, et al. Novel stem/progenitor cell population from murine tracheal submucosal gland ducts with multipotent regenerative potential. Stem Cells 2011;29: 1283–93.
16. Rock JR, Randell SH, Hogan BL. Airway basal stem cells: a perspective on their roles in epithelial homeostasis and remodelling. Dis Model Mech 2010; 3:545–56.
17. Epstein SK. Anatomy and physiology of tracheostomy. Respir Care 2005;50:476–82.
18. Kandjov IM. Heat and water rate transfer processes in the human respiratory tract at various altitudes. J Theor Biol 2001;208:287–93.
19. Sedlacek B. Die Befeuchtungsleistung hydrophober Heat und Moisture Exchanger (HME) unter klinischen Bedingungen. Dissertation. Charité – Universitätsmedizin Berlin. Berlin: Klinik für Anästhesiologie und Operative Intensivmedizin; 2006.
20. Finkbeiner WE. Physiology and pathology of tracheobronchial glands. Respir Physiol 1999;118: 77–83.
21. van der Schans CP. Bronchial mucus transport. Respir Care 2007;52:1150–6.
22. Nishino T, Hiraga K, Tadanobu M, et al. Respiratory reflex responses to stimulation of tracheal mucosa in enflurane-anesthetized humans. J Appl Phys 1988; 65:1069–74.

Pathology of Tracheal Tumors

Klaus Junker

KEYWORDS

• Tracheal tumors • Pathology • Squamous cell carcinoma • Adenoid cystic carcinoma
• Epithelial precursor lesions

KEY POINTS

- In general, patients with tracheal malignancies show an unfavorable prognosis with reported 5- and 10-year survival rates of 5% to 15% and 6% to 7%, respectively, for all types of tracheal carcinoma.
- The most important prognostic factors in primary malignant diseases of the trachea are early diagnosis, tumor stage, histology, and treatment options.
- Because of their predominantly local growth pattern, malignant salivary gland–type tumors show a better outcome than other histologic types.
- Surgical cure of adenoid cystic carcinoma may be impossible because of its characteristic relentless growth along the perineural sheath.
- Survival in patients with resectable tumors is better than in nonresected patients, especially after histologically complete resection.
- Selection of patients for definitive surgery is the most important factor in improving the prognosis for patients with primary tracheal malignancies.

The trachea extends from the lower border of the cricoid cartilage to the carina, averaging a length of 11 to 12 cm in adults.[1] Malignant involvement of the trachea predominantly results from direct spread of neighboring tumors, whereas primary tracheal malignancies are rarely observed.

EPIDEMIOLOGY

In adults, approximately 90% of all primary tumors of the trachea are malignant, in contrast to 10% to 30% in children. The incidence of tracheal malignancies is about 0.1 in every 100,000 persons per year, corresponding to approximately 0.2% of all tumors of the respiratory tract and to 0.02% to 0.04% of all malignant tumors. Malignancies of the larynx and bronchi are about 40 and 400 times more frequently observed than cancers of the trachea, respectively.[2,3]

Squamous cell carcinoma and adenoid cystic carcinoma make up about two-thirds of adult primary tracheal tumors. A heterogeneous group of benign and malignant tumors accounts for the remaining third of tracheal neoplasms (see next section).[4]

WORLD HEALTH ORGANIZATION CLASSIFICATION

There is no separate histologic classification for tracheal neoplasms. Primary tumors of the trachea are not listed in the World Health Organization (WHO) classification of tumors of the lung, pleura, thymus, and heart, but are summarized in the WHO classification of head and neck tumors, together with neoplasms of the hypopharynx and larynx. In the histologic classification of tumors of the hypopharynx, larynx, and trachea, malignant epithelial tumors (including several variants of squamous cell carcinoma as well as malignant salivary gland–type tumors), neuroendocrine tumors, benign epithelial tumors, soft-tissue tumors (benign and malignant), hematolymphoid tumors, tumors of bone and cartilage, mucosal malignant melanomas, and secondary tumors are listed.[5] Most of these neoplasms occur in the hypopharynx

Institute of Pathology, Bremen Central Hospital, St. Juergen-Strasse 1, Bremen 28177, Germany
E-mail address: klaus.junker@klinikum-bremen-mitte.de

Thorac Surg Clin 24 (2014) 7–11
http://dx.doi.org/10.1016/j.thorsurg.2013.09.008
1547-4127/14/$ – see front matter

or larynx, whereas only a low incidence is observed in the trachea.

TNM CLASSIFICATION

There is no generally accepted TNM classification for tracheal malignancies.[6] Because of the rareness of these tumors there are only proposed staging systems for primary tracheal carcinomas, which are not based on a large number of considered cases. To date their effectiveness has not been investigated prospectively.[4,7,8] Consequently, the application of a staging system for tracheal malignancies cannot be generally recommended.

Nevertheless, today a TNM classification can be used to allow a standardized description of the extent of tracheal malignancies. For this purpose, **Table 1** shows a modification of the staging system proposed by Macchiarini[4] in 2006, adapted to the general rules of the TNM system according to the seventh edition of the TNM classification of malignant tumors.[6]

PREMALIGNANT LESIONS

According to the WHO classification, epithelial precursor lesions are defined as altered epithelium with an increased likelihood for progression to squamous cell carcinoma. The 2005 WHO classification distinguishes between squamous cell hyperplasia, mild dysplasia, moderate dysplasia, severe dysplasia, and carcinoma in situ. In the SIN (squamous intraepithelial neoplasia) concept, mild dysplasia corresponds to SIN1 and moderate dysplasia to SIN2, whereas severe dysplasia and

Table 1
TNM staging system for primary tracheal malignancies

T	Primary Tumor
Tx	Primary tumor cannot be assessed
T0	No evidence of primary tumor
Tis	Carcinoma in situ
T1a	<3 cm, limited to the mucosa
T1b	≥3 cm, limited to the mucosa
T2	Invasion of cartilage or adventitia
T3	Invasion of larynx, carina or main bronchus
T4	Invasion of other neighboring structures
N	Lymph Nodes
Nx	Regional lymph nodes cannot be assessed
N0	No evidence of regional lymph node metastasis
N1	Local lymph node metastasis
Upper third	Highest mediastinal, upper paratracheal, prevascular and retrotracheal lymph nodes
Middle third	Upper paratracheal, prevascular and retrotracheal, lower paratracheal, para-aortic (ascending aorta or phrenic) lymph nodes
Lower third	Upper paratracheal, prevascular and retrotracheal, subaortic (aortopulmonary window) lymph nodes
N1a	1–3 lymph node metastasis
N1b	>3 lymph node metastasis
N2	Regional lymph node metastasis
Upper third	Lower paratracheal, subaortic (aortopulmonary window) lymph nodes
Middle third	Highest mediastinal, subaortic (aortopulmonary window) lymph nodes
Lower third	Upper paratracheal, pulmonary ligament lymph nodes
M	Distant Metastasis
M0	No evidence of distant metastasis
M1	Distant metastasis
M1a	Metastasis to lymph nodes other than N1 and N2
M1b	Distant metastasis

Modified from Macchiarini P. Primary tracheal tumours. Lancet Oncol 2006;7:83–91; with permission.

carcinoma in situ are not separated and are categorized as SIN3.[5]

The etiology of these premalignant lesions is strongly associated with tobacco smoking.[5] To date there has been no convincing evidence that human papillomavirus (HPV) infection plays a decisive role in the etiology of the epithelial precursor lesions of the trachea, whereas the majority, if not all cases of multiple airway papillomas are caused by HPV (**Fig. 1**). In 3% to 5% of these papillomas, progression to squamous cell carcinoma can be observed.[9]

SQUAMOUS CELL CARCINOMA

Squamous cell carcinoma is one of the most frequent primary tracheal tumors, comprising about one-third of all tracheal neoplasms. In the 2005 WHO classification, several variants of squamous cell carcinoma of the hypopharynx, larynx, and trachea are mentioned, including verrucous carcinoma, basaloid carcinoma, papillary carcinoma, spindle-cell carcinoma, acantholytic carcinoma, and adenosquamous carcinoma.[5]

Macroscopically, tracheal squamous cell carcinoma usually grows as a polypoid and frequently ulcerative mass, projecting into the lumen of the trachea.[5,10] In symptomatic stages, most of these lesions are easily detectable by bronchoscopy. Histologically these tumors are characterized by more or less well defined squamous differentiation, with or without keratinization (**Fig. 2**). The etiology of squamous cell carcinoma of the trachea is identical to that of the epithelial precursor lesions already described. The association with cigarette smoking may lead to metachronous or synchronous lesions of the oropharynx, the larynx, or the lungs.

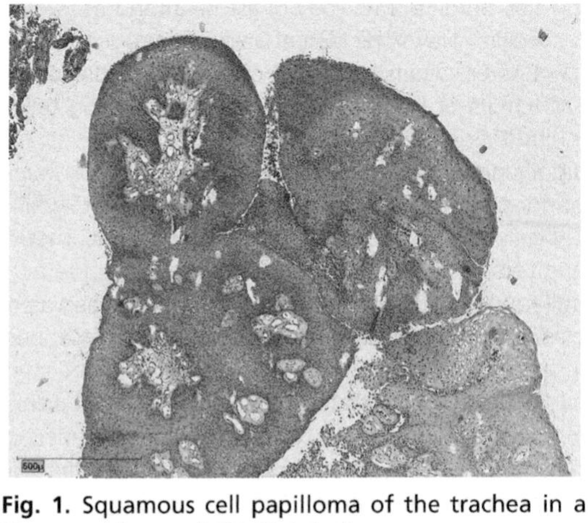

Fig. 1. Squamous cell papilloma of the trachea in a 77-year-old man. (H&E Staining).

MALIGNANT SALIVARY GLAND–TYPE TUMORS

Adenoid Cystic Carcinoma

Together with squamous cell carcinoma, adenoid cystic carcinoma represents the most frequent type of primary tracheal neoplasms, accounting for approximately another third of all tumors of the trachea.[3]

According to the WHO classification, adenoid cystic carcinoma is defined as a basaloid tumor consisting of epithelial and myoepithelial cells in variable morphologic configurations including tubular, cribriform, and solid patterns (**Fig. 3**).[5]

Macroscopically, tracheal adenoid cystic carcinoma usually shows exophytic nodular growth, leading to stenosis of the lumen of the trachea. Histologically these tumors consist of 2 main cell types: ductal (luminal) and myoepithelial (abluminal) cells. Local perineural spread is a hallmark of adenoid cystic carcinoma, with a tendency to develop recurrent disease after surgical resection (**Fig. 4**). The etiology of these neoplasms is unknown. In contrast to squamous cell carcinoma, adenoid cystic carcinomas are not associated with tobacco smoking.[5,11]

Secondary Tumors

Metastases to the tracheal wall are very unusual events. Most of these metastatic tumors are associated with far advanced stages of malignant diseases. Sites of corresponding primary tumors may be the breast, the colon, or the skin (melanomas).[5,12,13] Continuous spread to the trachea is much more frequently observed, emanating from thyroid carcinoma, esophageal carcinoma, lung cancer, thymic malignancies, or metastatic mediastinal lymph nodes.

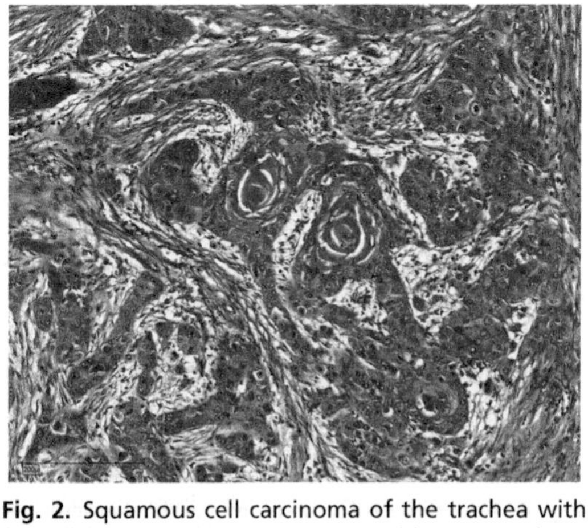

Fig. 2. Squamous cell carcinoma of the trachea with focal keratinization in a 61-year-old woman. (H&E Staining).

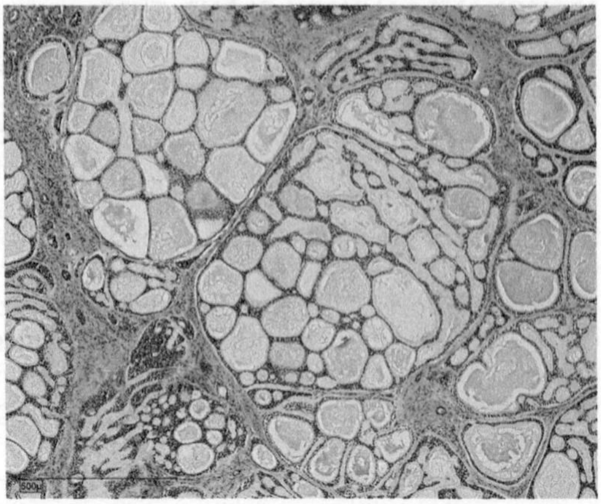

Fig. 3. Adenoid cystic carcinoma of the trachea with cribriform pattern in a 44-year-old man. (H&E Staining).

Prognosis

In general, patients with tracheal malignancies show an unfavorable prognosis, with reported 5- and 10-year survival rates of 5% to 15% and 6% to 7%, respectively, for all types of tracheal carcinoma.[3]

The most important prognostic factors in primary malignant diseases of the trachea are early diagnosis, tumor stage, histology, and treatment options.[2,7,14,15] Because of their predominantly local growth pattern, malignant salivary gland–type tumors show a better outcome in comparison with other histologic types. However, surgical cure of adenoid cystic carcinoma may be impossible because of its characteristic relentless growth along the perineural sheath. Nevertheless, survival in patients with resectable tumors is better than in nonresected patients, especially after histologically complete resection. Thus, selection of patients for definitive surgery is the most important factor in improving the prognosis for patients with primary tracheal malignancies.[2,3,16]

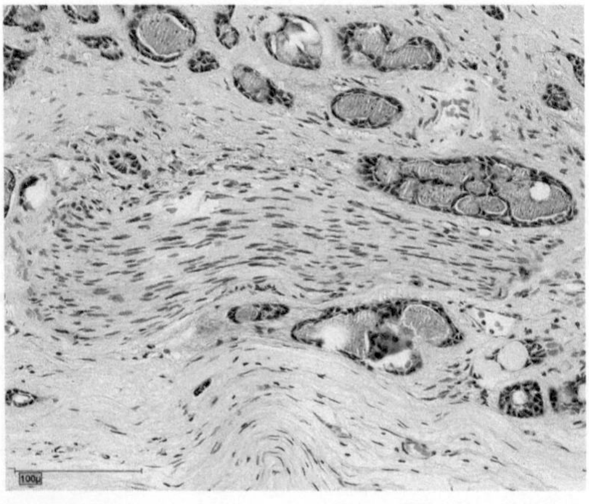

Fig. 4. Adenoid cystic carcinoma with characteristic growth along perineural sheath in an 80-year-old man. (H&E Staining).

REFERENCES

1. Mathisen DJ, Grillo HC. Tumors of the cervical trachea. In: Myers EN, Suen JY, editors. Cancer of the head and neck. 3rd edition. Philadelphia: WB Saunders; 1996. p. 439–61.
2. Honings J, van Dijck JA, Verhagen AF, et al. Incidence and treatment of tracheal cancer: a nationwide study in the Netherlands. Ann Surg Oncol 2007;14:968–76.
3. Honings J, Gaissert HA, van der Heijden HF, et al. Clinical aspects and treatment of primary tracheal malignancies. Acta Otolaryngol 2010;130:763–72.
4. Macchiarini P. Primary tracheal tumours. Lancet Oncol 2006;7:83–91.
5. Barnes L, Eveson JW, Reichart P, et al, editors. WHO classification of tumours, pathology and genetics, head and neck tumours. Lyon (France): IARC Press; 2005. p. 107–62.
6. Sobin L, Gospodarowicz M, Wittekind C, editors. TNM classification of malignant tumours. 7th edition. Oxford (United Kingdom): Wiley-Blackwell; 2009.
7. Licht PB, Friis S, Pettersson G. Tracheal cancer in Denmark: a nationwide study. Eur J Cardiothorac Surg 2001;19:339–45.
8. Bhattacharyya N. Contemporary staging and prognosis for primary tracheal malignancies: a population-based analysis. Otolaryngol Head Neck Surg 2004;131:639–42.
9. Odata-Suetsuga S, Izumi M, Takayama K, et al. A case of multiple squamous cell papillomas of the trachea. Ann Thorac Cardiovasc Surg 2011;17:212–4.
10. Heffner DK. Diseases of the trachea. In: Barnes L, editor. Surgical pathology of the head and neck. 2nd edition. New York: Marcel Dekker; 2001. p. 602–31.
11. Ellis GL, Auclair PL. AFIP atlas of tumor pathology, tumors of the salivary glands. Silver Spring (MD): ARP Press; 2008.
12. Conti JA, Kemeny N, Klimstra D, et al. Colon carcinoma metastatic to the trachea. Report of a case and review of the literature. Am J Clin Oncol 1994;17:227–9.
13. Koyi H, Branden E. Intratracheal metastasis from malignant melanoma. J Eur Acad Dermatol Venereol 2000;14:407–8.
14. Gaissert HA, Grillo HC, Shadmehr MB, et al. Long-term survival after resection of primary adenoid cystic and squamous cell carcinoma of the trachea and the carina. Ann Thorac Surg 2004;78:1889–97.

15. Yang KY, Chen YM, Huang MH, et al. Revisit of primary malignant neoplasms of the trachea: clinical characteristics and survival analysis. Jpn J Clin Oncol 1997;27:305–9.
16. Li Y, Peng A, Yang X, et al. Clinical manifestation and management of primary malignant tumors of the cervical trachea. Eur Arch Otorhinolaryngol 2013. [Epub ahead of print].

Anesthesia and Gas Exchange in Tracheal Surgery

Klaus Wiedemann*, Clemens Männle

KEYWORDS

• Tracheal stenosis • Airway tumors • Airway management • Ventilation techniques • Bronchoscopy

KEY POINTS

- Gas exchange across the open airways in tracheobronchial surgery (TBS) is commonly maintained either by intubation over the surgical field or by jet ventilation through a small-bore catheter into the severed airway. Cross-field intubation-ventilation is a fallback procedure throughout TBS.
- Apneic oxygenation is a rare method of gas exchange during intricate airway surgery. Extracorporeal lung support may be indicated in anticipated loss of airway viability during induction of anesthesia or in extensive TBS.
- Command by the anesthesiologist of fiberoptic bronchoscopy is indispensible for airway management in tracheobronchial disorders and for close communication with the surgeon.
- Tracheal surgery poses unique challenges for airway management in critical obstruction. Nature, location, and extent of the tracheal disorder determine choice of anesthetic induction and airway access. On ill-timed extubation with residual opioid and relaxant effects or subglottic edema, airway viability may rapidly be lost. A decision on supportive medication, reintubation, or emergency tracheostomy must quickly be arrived at.

INTRODUCTION

In tracheobronchial surgery (TBS) sharing the airways with the surgeon and carrying the main responsibility for airway access and respiratory function are challenges for the anesthesiologist. The methods of gas exchange used differ at first glance from customary ventilation but, based on physics and physiology, they constitute safe procedures. Understanding of causative disorders and their impacts on airway patency during anesthetic induction, of surgery, and the consequences of airway reconstruction for emergence and postoperative care must combine to provide consistent management. Command of fiberoptic bronchoscopy (FOB) and swift reaction to emergencies are required to preserve airway viability. Ventilation techniques and airway control are based largely on accumulated experience; because of the moderate incidence of TBS, there are few studies to establish evidence beyond expert opinion. Recent surgical developments require open-minded sharing of airways and ideas.

TECHNIQUES OF GAS EXCHANGE DURING TBS

Jet Ventilation

Definition

Jet ventilation (JV) means the pulsed delivery of volumes of gas from a high-pressure source across small-bore catheters. Because of the

Disclosures: K. Wiedemann received remuneration of travel expenses for scientific meetings from ACUTRONIC Medical Systems AG, CH-8816 Hirzel/Switzerland. As corresponding author of a video on high-frequency jet ventilation commissioned by ACUTRONIC Medical Systems AG, CH-8816 Hirzel/Switzerland, and IfM Ingenieurbüro für Medizintechnik GmbH, D - 35435 Wettenberg, Germany, he received remuneration of travel expenses. C. Männle has no direct financial interest in the subject matter or materials discussed in the article or with a company making a competing product.

Department of Anesthesiology and Intensive Care, Thoraxklinik, University Hospitals, Amalienstr.5, Heidelberg D-69126, Germany
* Corresponding author. Panoramastr.103, Heidelberg D-69126, Germany.
E-mail address: wiedemann.panorama.hd@t-online.de

Thorac Surg Clin 24 (2014) 13–25
http://dx.doi.org/10.1016/j.thorsurg.2013.10.001
1547-4127/14/$ – see front matter

thoracic.theclinics.com

kinetic energy imparted, the gas portions travel into the airways independently of the airways' integrity and of any airtight connection to the ventilator (loose coupling). Low-frequency JV (LFJV) (20–60 cycles/min) is delivered by manual devices, and high-frequency JV (HFJV) (60–600 cycles/min) by purpose-built ventilators. With increasing frequency, tidal excursions of the respiratory system are diminished. Thus the main attractions of HFJV in TBS are loose coupling, facilitated surgical access by small-diameter jet catheters, and a quiet surgical field from low tidal excursions.

Respiratory physiology in HFJV

Gas exchange with tidal volumes (v_t) smaller than dead space (v_D) mainly depends on continuous laminar flow in the small airways, with the injected gas traveling in the center, and the expiratory gas along the bronchial walls.[1]

Parameters

Pressures Driving pressure (DP), from 0.5 to 4.0 atm, is selected at the reducing valve in the jet ventilator. It is the main determinant of v_t. Airway pressure (AwP) is the pressure resulting from the v_t delivered into the airways, and the properties of the respiratory system. Peak AwP is less than in conventional ventilation.[2]

Volumes The v_t delivered by the jet ventilator mainly results from DP and from the resistance of the jet catheter. The vt introduced into the airways depends on respiratory impedance, entrainment, and spillage from the airway.[3] Entrainment of ambient air at the catheter orifice, if located in the trachea, is low.[3,4] However, resultant dilution of fraction of oxygen in the gas delivered by the jet ventilator as preselected (Fjet O_2) may reduce inspiratory oxygen concentration (FiO_2) in the airways.

Δ Fjet O_2 1.0 should be selected throughout.

For settings and handling of HFJV during TBS, see section HFJV on the page 19.

Concerns with jet ventilation

Barotrauma The high gas flows delivered during inspiration cannot be accommodated by the respiratory system. Any impedance to continuous egress of gas from the airways causes a dangerous increase in AwP within a few jet cycles, promoting barotrauma.[4]

Δ Egress of gas from the airways during jet ventilation must never be impeded.

Jet ventilators, but not manual devices, at preselected pressure thresholds cut off ventilation (**Figs. 1–3**).[5–7] In laryngeal surgery, use of manual

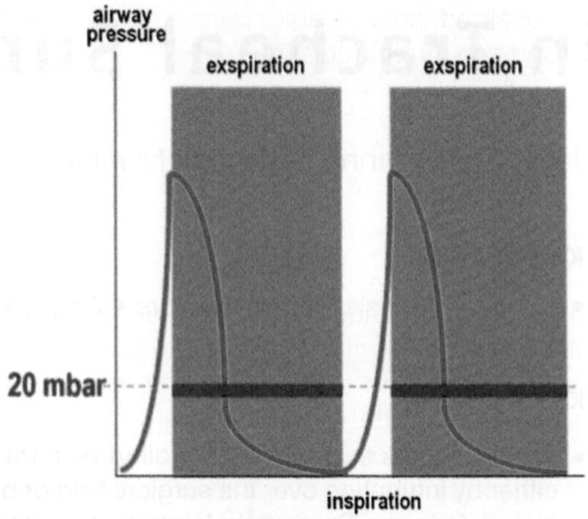

Fig. 1. Pressure monitoring and safety features in high-frequency jet ventilators. Pause pressure (PP) is sensed for the last 10 milliseconds of expiratory pause. If PP fails to undercut the 20 mbar threshold, cycling is blocked. Cycling is resumed when PP has decreased to less than 20% of threshold value. Incremental increase of AwPs from volume stacking is prevented. (*Courtesy of* P. Biro, MD, Institute of Anesthesiology, University Hospital, Zurich, Switzerland.)

jet devices, or continuing HFJV despite outflow obstruction, has caused 3 deaths[8] or severe complications from barotrauma.[8,9] In TBS, barotrauma from HFJV has not been reported.[10,11]

Hypothermia and exsiccation The jet gas is cooled by decompression at the jet nozzle. Thus the respiratory system loses heat and moisture. Some jet ventilators provide gas conditioning at 37°C.[7]

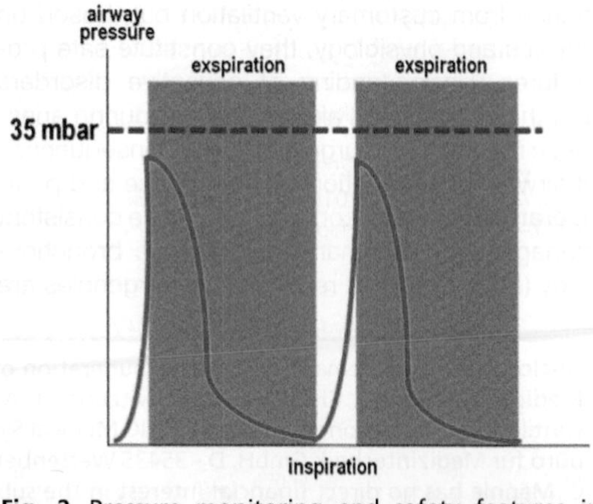

Fig. 2. Pressure monitoring and safety features in high-frequency jet ventilators. AwP is sensed continuously through the dedicated channel of a double-lumen jet catheter. If peak inspiratory pressure exceeds the preselected 35-mbar threshold, the ventilator is cut off. (*Courtesy of* P. Biro, MD, Institute of Anesthesiology, University Hospital, Zurich, Switzerland.)

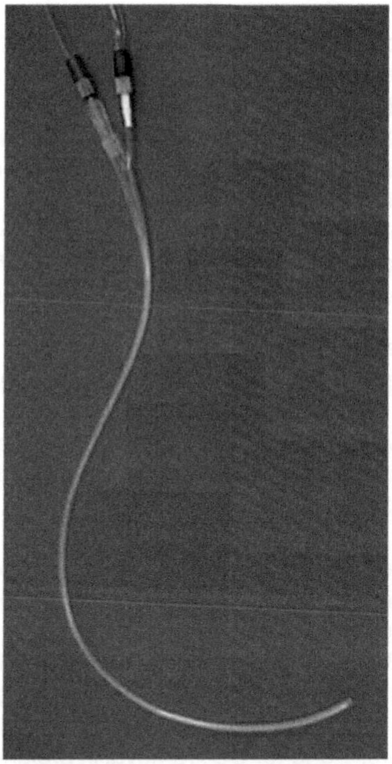

Fig. 3. Pressure monitoring and safety features in high-frequency jet ventilators. Double-lumen jet catheter (Aerojet, Dahlhausen, Cologne, Germany). The blue connector designates the channel for jet ventilation and sensing of PP. The red connector designates the monitoring channel for continuous sensing of AwP.

Apneic Oxygenation

Definition

Apneic oxygenation (AO) relies on the physiologic oxygen stores of the body and on apneic mass movement to meet oxygen demand during interruption of ventilation.

Physiologic considerations

Oxygen Pulmonary oxygen stores in the adult with a functional residual capacity (FRC) of 3000 mL on total washout of nitrogen by preoxygenation contains 2650 mL (88.6 vol%). This process is 95% completed during normal ventilation after 3 minutes. The intrapulmonary oxygen store meets an oxygen demand during anesthesia of 200 mL/min for more than 10 minutes.[12,13] The diffusion balance of gases involved, N_2, CO_2, and O_2 across open airways causes a net inflow to the alveoli. This apneic mass movement[14,15] with insufflation of oxygen (10–12 L/min) is the basic mechanism for sustained oxygenation during apnea.

Carbon dioxide and respiratory acidosis $Paco_2$ may increase by 10 to 13 mm Hg[16] during the first minute of apnea and 3 to 4 mm Hg/min[17] thereafter. After 15 minutes, $Paco_2$ was 73.2 ± 9.9 mm Hg at mean pH 7.2 in 31 subjects,[18] and after 53 minutes was 250 mm Hg at pH 6.72.[19] No buffers were administered, and uneventful recovery was reported. Buffering in respiratory acidosis is discussed elsewhere.[20,21]

Hypercapnia and effects on circulation In moderate hypercapnia, blood pressure tends to increase with an increase in cardiac output and reduction of peripheral resistance.[22] Arrhythmias during AO occur to varying degrees.[18,19] Because cerebral blood flow may increase to 4 mL/100 g × min/mm Hg $Paco_2$,[23] AO is contraindicated during episodes of augmented intracranial blood volume, such as from clamping the superior vena cava.[24]

Clinical aspects of AO

Episodic AO in TBS is common for intermittent removal of airways from the surgical site.[25] For delicate TBS, predetermined AO is thought to be decisive.[26] Prerequisites are complete nitrogen washout, and tracheal oxygen insufflation of 10 to 15 L/min for apneic mass movement. For AO at 60 minutes, mean $Paco_2$ was 105 mm Hg and Pao_2 117 mm Hg.[27] No hemodynamic reactions or neurologic disturbances were observed.[24,27] Contraindications to AO are significant coronary artery disease, pulmonary arterial hypertension, chronic hypoxemia, and increased intracranial volume. In obesity AO is contraindicated because of the diminished FRC.[18,28]

Airway Surgery in the Awake Patient

Extrathoracic airway surgery in the awake under cervical extradural anesthesia (CEA) may offer advantages.[29] As endotracheal airways are dispensable, surgical exposure is unobstructed. Reconstruction is facilitated by unimpaired vocal cord observation and preserved patient communication. Recovery may be accelerated by unimpaired cough reflex, early ambulation, and early oral intake.

General aspects of CEA

CEA has been used predominantly for carotid surgery[30] (for detailed discussion see Refs.[30–32]). An epidural catheter is inserted at the C6 to C7 or C7 to T1 vertebral interspaces, observing common precautions. Choice and concentrations of anesthetic agents are directed at the avoidance of motor blockade.[29,32] Sensory blockade from C2 to T8 involving the cervical superficial plexus (C1–C4) and brachial superficial plexus (C5–T8) for each segment requires 1.5 mL of anesthetic.[30] Functions and regions not affected by CEA, include the laryngeal nerves, which derive from the vagus nerve and are not blocked, so vocal cord activity is preserved. CEA in surgery involving the pharyngotracheal region, requires supplemental local anesthesia for blockade of vagal afferents.[29,31]

Physiologic effects of CEA

Sympathetic blockade by CEA induces moderate bradycardia and slight hypotension. Myocardial oxygen consumption is reduced.[31] Laryngeal pressure responses to laryngoscopy and intubation from vagal afferents are preserved. Circulatory responses to stimulation of the bronchocarinal region are suppressed from blockade of sympathetic afferents.[33] Respiratory effects produce a restrictive pattern of pulmonary function. Diminution of dynamic lung volumes suggests compromise of cough strength and bronchial clearance.[34,35]

Experience in CEA for extrathoracic tracheal surgery

Anesthetic management in 20 awake patients comprised CEA with repetitive doses of ropivacaine and intraoperatively atomizing mepivacaine onto pretracheal structures to prevent coughing.[29] Verbal communication was well maintained, as was oxygenation by mask and intratracheal insufflation. (It is one of the advantages of tracheal surgery in the awake that verbal communication is maintained and assessment of resectable trachea length is facilitated.) Comparable infralaryngeal exposure and early recovery are also achieved by prudent selection of airways (see section Jet Ventilation, and section Anesthesia and Ventilation in Extrathoracic Tracheal Resection; **Figs. 5–7**) and intravenous anesthesia. Complication rates in CEA for carotid surgery[30,32] are in the range of those for thoracic epidural anesthesia,[36,37] except for more than double the rate for subarachnoid injection.[32]

Extracorporeal Gas Exchange in TBS

Cardiopulmonary bypass

Cardiopulmonary bypass (CPB) affords oxygenation and stable hemodynamics. Disadvantages such as increased hemorrhage from anticoagulation, systemic inflammation from traumatized blood components, and propensity to acute lung injury are detailed elsewhere.[38,39] CPB is used in cancer surgery involving central airways and cardiovascular structures,[38] or in airway compromise for bridging gas exchange between anesthetic induction and surgical airway access.[40]

Extracorporeal membrane oxygenation

In extracorporeal membrane oxygenation (ECMO), centrifugal or axial pumps, a membrane oxygenator, and lack of a blood reservoir reduce blood component trauma and release of inflammatory mediators.[39,41,42] Thus venoarterial ECMO, in providing total gas exchange and stable circulation, is replacing CPB for combined central airway and cardiovascular procedures.[39,43] CPB is still indispensable in cancer surgery involving heart and central vessels.[44] Venovenous ECMO is not intended for full circulatory support, but provides gas exchange in emergency procedures for central airway rupture[45] or tracheal obstruction.[46]

Pumpless interventional lung assist

Pumpless interventional lung assist (iLA) comprises an artificial arteriovenous shunt with a low-resistance membrane gas exchanger interconnected. Blood flow depends on the arteriovenous pressure difference, requiring a mean arterial pressure greater than 70 mm Hg. The main indication for iLA is CO_2 removal and correction of respiratory acidosis. Its potential for oxygen transfer is limited.[47]

In TBS, iLA has been used for CO_2 elimination in protective ventilation for acute lung injury during repair of tracheobronchial or pulmonary disorders,[48] and for CO_2 removal in prolonged apnea during delicate surgery.[44,48,49] Apneic periods up to 10 hours[49] with normocapnia were achieved.[44,48] Preoxygenation and tracheal O_2 insufflation are indispensible for oxygenation (see section Apneic Oxygenation). Complications of iLA are about 10% from venous and 8% from arterial long-term access.[42] Intraoperative hypothermia may occur.[48]

CLINICAL PROCEDURES IN ANESTHESIA FOR TBS

General Aspects of Anesthesia and Gas Exchange in Tracheobronchial Surgery

It is important to understand the exponential correlation between airway diameter and degree of respiratory compromise (**Box 1**).

Diagnostics

From the patient's history the least distressful body position indicates the position best suited to maintain a viable airway during anesthetic induction. The extent of tracheal stenosis is reflected by the degree of obstructive respiratory dysfunction with diminished FEV_1 (forced expiratory volume in 1 second). Flow-volume loops in pulmonary function tests (PFTs) may indicate the degree, position, and nature of the stenosis. FOB or rigid bronchoscopy affords evaluation of the lesion regarding its position relative to the larynx and its longitudinal and intraluminal extension. The nature of the process, either fixed or malacic (variable), can be assessed. In fixed stenoses,

Box 1
Clinical considerations from the Hagen-Poiseuille laminar flow equation

$$\text{resistance} = \frac{\text{pressure drop}}{\text{flow}} = \frac{8 \times \text{viscosity} \times \text{length}}{\pi \times \text{radius}^4}$$

1. Airway resistance increases 16 times when airway radius is halved
2. Rapid progression of symptoms with reduction of airway patency:
   - It takes a 50% reduction (to 8 mm) in adults for there to be symptoms at exertion
   - It needs a small reduction (to 5–6 mm) for there to be inspiratory stridor at rest
3. Impact on respiratory effort of swelling, secretions, airway instrumentation
4. Value of antiinflammatory medication, bronchoscopic dilation

Adapted from Hobai IA, Chhangani SV, Alfille PH. Anesthesia for tracheal resection and reconstruction. Anesthesiol Clin 2012;30:711–12; with permission.

preoperative dilation may improve perioperative airway patency.[50]

Conduct of anesthesia

Total intravenous anesthesia Total intravenous anesthesia is indispensible in the presence of a severed airway. Propofol as the hypnotic and remifentanil as the opioid, and short-acting muscular relaxants such as mivacurium are applied. The α-2 adrenergic agonist dexmedetomidine produces anxiolysis, sedation, and analgesia without respiratory depression. Dexmedetomidine can replace inhalational anesthesia for induction and airway management when preservation of spontaneous respiration is required in severe stenosis.[51–53] It may facilitate controlled emergence.[25,54]

Inhalational anesthetics Induction with sevoflurane inhalational anesthesia is advocated when maintained spontaneous respiration is crucial in severe stenosis for preservation of residual airway viability. Airway manipulation during light anesthesia may provoke coughing or laryngospasm and loss of airway patency. Dexmedetomidine does not produce comparable reactions and so may be preferable.

Anesthetic induction in critical airway stenosis In fixed stenosis, as in tracheal scars, intravenous induction and rapid-action muscular relaxation is appropriate. Manual positive pressure ventilation (PPV) improves airflow across the restriction.[55] In variable extrathoracic stenosis (eg, tracheomalacia), PPV counteracts inspiratory collapse, and conventional induction is used. For variable intrathoracic stenosis, as from tracheomalacia or pedunculated tumors, anesthetic induction under spontaneous respiration is advocated because of concern for tracheal collapse from increased intrathoracic pressure during PPV.[56] Successful attempts at manual ventilation in the unresponsive patient permit muscular relaxation for intubation. Otherwise insertion must be accomplished in deep anesthesia under spontaneous respiration, direct laryngoscopy, and FOB guidance. Rescue plans for failed intubation comprise HFJV across a rigid bronchoscope or transtracheally, ensuring unimpeded expiratory outflow (see section Jet Ventilation), surgical airway access, or using variants of extracorporeal gas exchange (see section Extracorporeal Gas Exchange in TBS).

Pain therapy

In extrathoracic airway surgery, low-potency opioids (eg, piritramide) applied by patient-controlled administration, and peripherally acting analgesics, provide pain control.

For intrathoracic airway surgery, whenever feasible thoracic epidural analgesia is initiated by awake catheter insertion at the T4 to T10 level and started before skin incision. Postoperative analgesia is supplemented with nonsteroidal Anti-inflammatory drugs (NSAIDs). Catheter-based paravertebral blockade is an alternative.[57] Both techniques may be used for 5 to 7 days under pain service supervision, followed by oral opioids and NSAIDs.

Monitoring and equipment

Standard noninvasive monitoring including anesthesia depth and neuromuscular transmission[58] is augmented by left radial artery cannulation for blood gas analyses, and by monitoring transcutaneous P_{CO_2} and core temperature. Forced air warming is routine.[59] In thoracotomies, additional vascular access comprises a central venous catheter and large-bore cannulas. A urinary catheter is inserted.

FOB FOB for the anesthetist is a prerequisite in airway management and monitoring of surgery. Thorough knowledge of endoscopic anatomy and close communication with the surgeon are indispensible. Equipment on site comprises customary FOBs for diagnostics and treatment, and dedicated intubation FOBs featuring an insertion tube of extended working length, enhanced rigidity, and outer diameter ~3 mm. Pediatric FOBs are inadequate. A rigid bronchoscope and a video laryngoscope are provided.

Airway management provisions The anesthetist's airway management provisions comprise supraglottic airways (laryngeal mask airway [LMA]), armored and plain endotracheal tubes (ETT), tracheal cannulas, double-lumen tubes (DLT), dedicated endobronchial tubes (**Fig. 8**), bronchial blockers (BBs; **Fig. 10**), and cannulas for transtracheal (jet)ventilation. Sterile surgical airway management provisions comprise airways for endotracheal or endobronchial cross-field intubation-ventilation (CFI–V) and a circuit for connection to the anesthesia ventilator.

Anesthesia and Ventilation in Extrathoracic Tracheal Resection

General considerations

Indications Most frequent indications are tracheal stenoses from intubation or tracheostomy.[60] Rare causes are malignancies, inflammation, and compression from adjacent structures (discussed by Welter and colleagues, Detterbeck and colleagues, and Macchiarini and Jungebluth elsewhere in this issue). For intraoperative ventilation, pressure-controlled ventilation (PCV) across an LMA or an ETT as a principal airway is used during tracheal dissection. With the trachea severed, gas exchange is maintained by HFJV through 12-Fr to 14-Fr double-lumen catheters (see **Fig. 3**) or by CFI-V.

HFJV

HFJV and alternatives HFJV is the recommended ventilation method for satisfactory surgical exposure (see section Jet Ventilation). If surgical intentions require an operative field devoid of any airway tubing, AO or spontaneous ventilation under CEA in the awake might be considered (see section Apneic Oxygenation, and section Airway Surgery in the Awake Patient). Extracorporeal gas exchange may be indicated, either when anesthesia or surgery might jeopardize ventilation with a trachea that is inaccessible to conventional intubation or in demanding surgical procedures (see section Extracorporeal Gas Exchange in TBS).

HFJV: technical considerations Principal airways as conduits for jet catheters are upraglottic or endotracheal.

LMA In using a supraglottic airway, commonly an LMA (**Fig. 4**),[61,62] infraglottic exposure is unimpeded by any length of ETT (see **Figs. 5–7**). In the standard LMA, the airway tube offers the largest diameter to concomitantly accommodate the jet catheter and an FOB. Because intubation of the larynx through a standard LMA is difficult, LMA and jet catheter are prearranged (see **Fig. 4**). In deep general and topical anesthesia under laryngoscopy, the jet catheter is guided into the trachea with its tip left above the stenotic area, and the LMA simultaneously brought to its supraglottic position.

Δ Do not attempt to pass the catheter tip across the stenosis

After insertion of LMA and jet catheter:

- By manual ventilation the LMA is tested for seal and unresisted inspiration and expiration
- The position of the catheter tip is checked by FOB

Δ Catheter tip must be above the stenosis

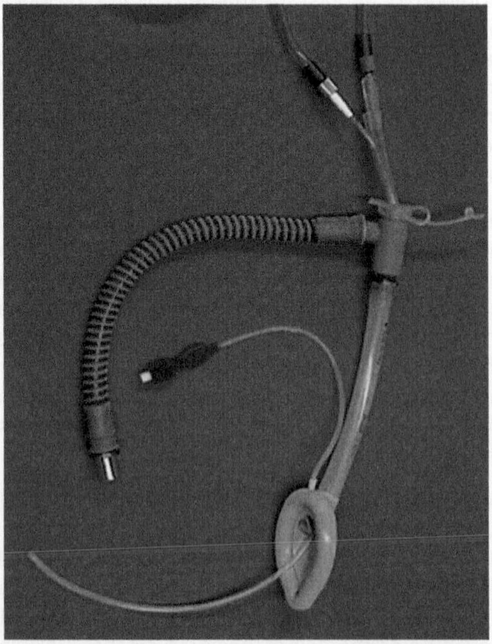

Fig. 4. Laryngeal Mask Airway (LMA) in tracheal surgery. A standard laryngeal mask (sLMA) (LMA North America Inc, San Diego, CA) is attached to the blue large-bore swivel connector with self-sealing diaphragm (Teleflex Medical, Kernen, Germany). A jet catheter has been inserted to protrude from the LMA's grille.

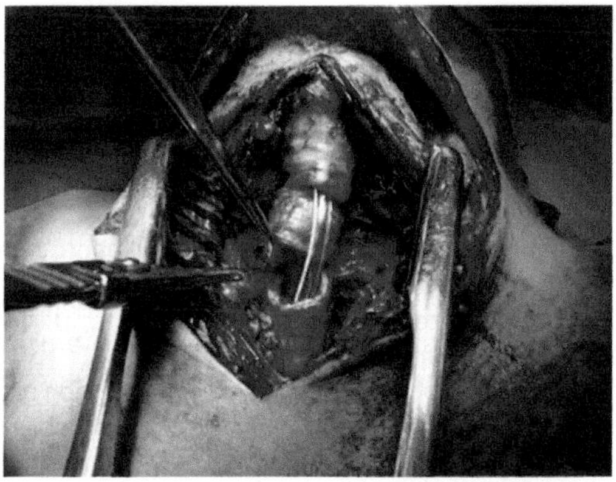

Fig. 5. HFJV during extrathoracic tracheal resection. A double-lumen jet catheter across an sLMA (cf **Fig. 4**) during induction of anesthesia was placed with its tip in the subcricoid region. After transection, in bypassing the stenotic segment the catheter has been advanced into the distal trachea for HFJV. (*Courtesy of* H. Hoffmann, MD, Thoraxklinik, Heidelberg, Germany.)

- If any condition is not attainable, the LMA is changed for an ETT
- With all conditions met, muscular relaxation is induced and PCV started

Δ At the start of HFJV, disconnect the LMA from the anesthesia circuit for free egress of expiratory gas

ETT An ETT of reasonable diameter should preferably pass the stenosis. If this proves unfeasible without undue force, the tip of the ETT is positioned closely above the stenosis. The short length of ETT remaining in the trachea is prone to inadvertent extubation.

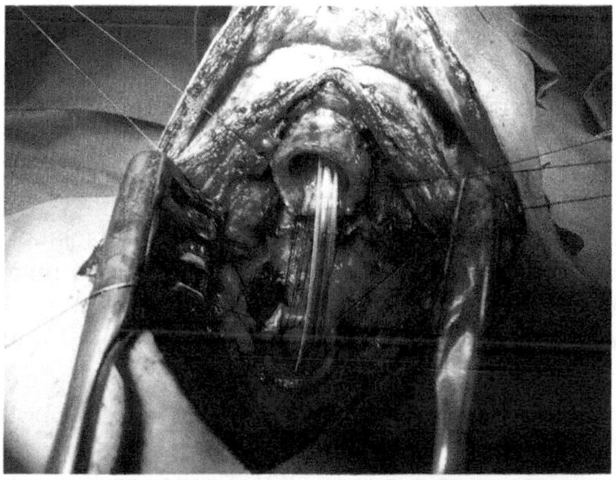

Fig. 6. HFJV during extrathoracic tracheal resection. Tracheal resection completed. Note unobstructed access to the infracricoid region during placement of sutures by use of the supraglottic airway as a conduit for the HFJV catheter (cf **Fig. 4**). (*Courtesy of* H. Hoffmann, MD, Thoraxklinik, Heidelberg, Germany.)

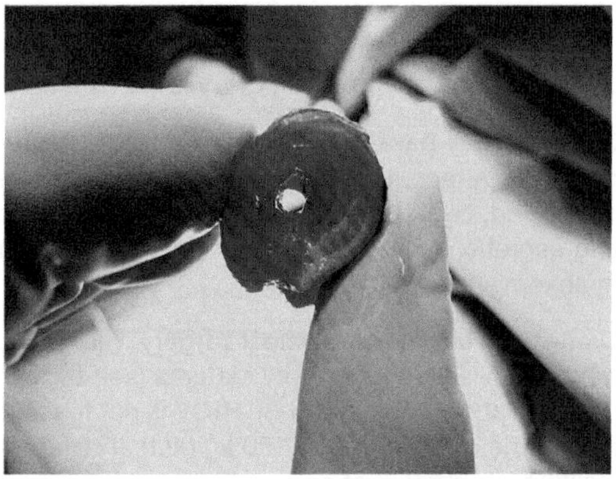

Fig. 7. HFJV during extrathoracic tracheal resection. The stenotic section leaves a tracheal lumen of less than 5 mm, precluding passage of a jet catheter and egress of expiratory gas during HFJV. Thus, before tracheal transection, the catheter tip had to be kept above the stenosis. (*Courtesy of* H. Hoffmann, MD, Thoraxklinik, Heidelberg, Germany.)

Tracheostomy cannula The cannula is preferably changed for transglottic intubation beyond the stoma. The ETT subsequently serves as a conduit for HFJV. If the intratracheal lesion precludes transglottic intubation, the tracheostomy cannula is used for PCV until tracheal transection. It is then changed for a jet catheter or an armored ETT for CFI-V.

Sequence of ventilation techniques During the dissection phase, conventional PCV with positive end-expiratory pressure (PEEP) of 6 mbar is used. Five minutes before transection of the trachea, preoxygenation with Fio_2 1.0 is commenced (see section Apneic Oxygenation). Once the trachea is opened, the jet catheter from the LMA or the ETT, or across the surgical field, is advanced caudad by the surgeon (see **Figs. 5–7**).

HFJV: settings and handling

- In the adult, DP is set to 20 mbar/kg body weight (bwt), cycling frequency (f) 100/min to 150/min, and Inspiratory/Expiratory time (I/E) ratio is 1.0. Fjet O_2 1.0 is selected (except in laser surgery).
- In hypercapnia, DP is increased by 0.4-bar increments to augment v_t. Large increases in DP eventually may cause volume stacking and intrinsic PEEP, due to the expiratory time becoming too short for the increased v_t to empty.
- In persistent hypercapnia and pH less than 7.1, CFI-V is instituted.
- In hypoxemia, endobronchial catheter malposition and accumulation of secretions are

treated first. Next, DP is increased as described earlier.

- In persistent hypoxemia, CFI-V is implemented.

CFI-V as a fall-back measure must always be prepared for. A recruitment maneuver should then be performed, because, with jet catheter malposition and secretions ruled out, the remaining cause for hypoxemia is atelectasis.

Limitations of HFJV in tracheal surgery HFJV may not be applied without safety features (see section Jet Ventilation; see **Figs. 1–3**). HFJV is not feasible in extreme obesity (120 to 150 kg bwt) and in preexisting impairment of gas exchange, when PEEP greater than 6 mbar and Fio_2 greater than 0.6 are required during PCV.

CFI-V

CFI-V is accomplished by having a sterile cuffed armored ETT inserted into the distal trachea by the surgeon. Ventilation is started across a sterile connection to the anesthesia circuit. Alternating as required by surgical exposure between CFI-V and extubation for intermittent apnea is customary. However, this is more tedious than using HFJV throughout, with CFI-V as the fall-back technique.

Termination of surgery and emergence from anesthesia

HFJV with completion of the tracheal anastomosis is tapered to a stop, the jet catheter is withdrawn, and PCV is resumed across the previously used LMA or ETT. In CFI-V with the membranous portion of the anastomosis accomplished, the cross-field tube is removed and the ETT formerly placed endotracheally is advanced with its cuff beyond the suture line, to complete the anastomosis under PCV.

Δ Preemergence FOB inspection serves to rule out; to identify; and, with clots or secretions present, to treat airway obstruction.

Emergence phase The patient should breathe spontaneously, and, with residual relaxation ruled out (Train-of-Four ratio near 0.9), the airway is removed. Preferably this is achieved in the operating room, where equipment for difficult airway management is readily available. Reintubation is best performed under FOB guidance and by direct laryngoscopy. A video laryngoscope may be helpful.[63]

Acute postoperative respiratory compromise Stabilization of airways by jaw thrust, insertion of oral or nasotracheal airways, and immediate oxygen administration by face mask and assisted ventilation are key steps. For rapid treatment, causes are identified concomitantly and the surgeon is informed.

1. Rule out or treat residual effects of anesthesia:
   Opioid effects produce bradypnea in a calm patient.
   Muscular relaxation produces agitation, respiratory distress, and flaccid muscle action.
   Antagonize as appropriate.
2. Rule out or treat airway obstruction:
   With symptoms of asphyxiation, insertion of a supraglottic airway (LMA) is attempted.
   If insertion and ventilation are successful, FOB identifies:
   - Infraglottic edema or bronchospasm amenable to treatment with epinephrine racemate or bronchodilators.
   - Obstruction at the anastomotic level amenable to removal of clots or secretions.
   - Vocal cord dysfunction necessitating intubation.
   - Obstruction requiring surgical action.

   If LMA insertion or ventilation fails, swift reintubation with FOB guidance is necessary before hypoxia sets in. In failed intubation, surgical airway access should not be delayed.

(*Adapted from* Ref.[56] with permission of the publisher and the author).

Postoperative care The patient is kept in an intensive care unit (ICU) or in intermediate care (IMC) for 24 hours (For pain therapy see section in the page 17).

Anesthesia and Ventilation for Sleeve Pneumonectomy and Carinal Resection

Surgical essentials

Details are discussed by Weder, and Hecker and colleagues elsewhere in this issue. Briefly, sleeve pneumonectomy involves the resection of 1 lung with parts of the lower trachea and of the contralateral main bronchus. After vascular isolation, the operative lung no longer contributes to right-to-left shunt during 1-lung ventilation (OLV). Carinal resection involves the partial removal of both main bronchi and of the lower trachea with subsequent reanastomosis. Because perfusion of both lungs is retained, right-to-left shunt and hypoxemia may occur during OLV. Ensnaring the right main pulmonary artery directs perfusion to the ventilated left lung to improve oxygenation.[64] Occasional bilateral ventilation must be prepared for by providing HFJV catheters or ETTs for bronchial insertion.

General aspects of anesthesia, pain therapy, and monitoring

See section General Aspects of Anesthesia and Gas Exchange in Tracheobronchial Surgery.

Management of airways and gas exchange

Sleeve pneumonectomy and carinal resection during surgical dissection require left-sided OLV. Results of preoperative bronchoscopy determine the choice of airways (see **Figs. 8–11**).

a. A DLT for left endobronchial intubation allows for differential recruiting techniques for the right lung.[65] Thus oxygenation during OLV can be preserved with right lung collapse tailored to surgical demand. Strict safety measures are adhered to. Position and extent of the lesion may preclude DLT use (**Box 2**, see **Fig. 9**).
b. Endobronchial intubation with a wire-reinforced endobronchial tube (WRETT) featuring a special cuff (see **Fig. 8**) is used for left-sided OLV.[25] FOB guidance is essential for positioning and management. Endobronchial intubation leaves the excluded lung inaccessible to any recruitment for oxygenation during impending hypoxemia short of 2-lung ventilation. Dislodgement often needs fiberoptic or surgical correction. Endobronchial intubation is also contraindicated in carinal lesions (see **Fig. 9**).
c. A BB across an ETT is advanced under FOB guidance into the right main bronchus. After positioning of the patient, BB position needs FOB confirmation to avoid damage to airways and intraluminal disorders. Only then may OLV to the left lung be instituted by inflating the cuff under FOB vision and cuff pressure monitoring (see **Figs. 10** and **11**). During impending hypoxemia, oxygen can be insufflated across the BB catheter into the right lung.

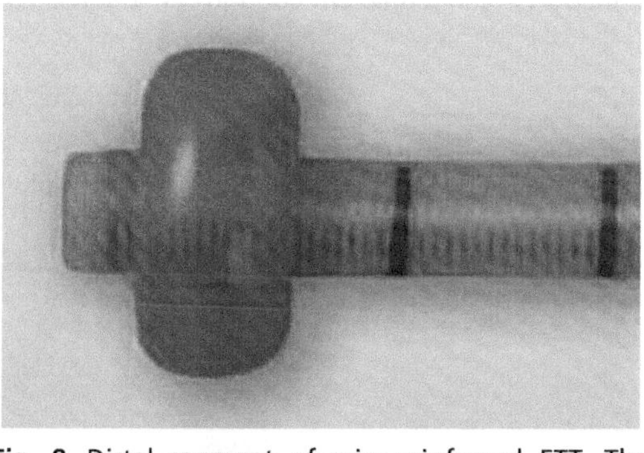

Fig. 8. Distal segment of wire-reinforced ETT. The doughnut-shaped cuff and the short tip afford shallow intubation of the main bronchus to avoid obstruction of lobar bronchial orifices. Permission for use granted by Fuji Systems Corporation, Tokyo, Japan.

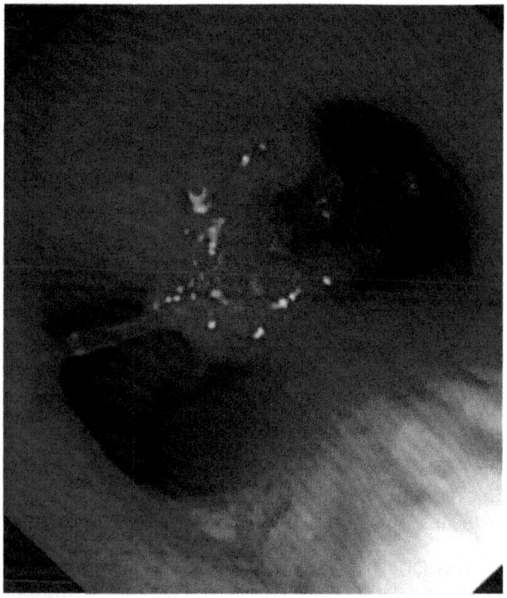

Fig. 9. BB for OLV: position in the main carina of this carcinoma precludes endobronchial intubation for OLV preceding carinal resection, necessitating BB use. (*Courtesy of* R. Eberhardt, MD, Thoraxklinik, Heidelberg, Germany.)

Ventilation techniques

Dissection phase OLV is instituted immediately before the thorax is entered, with F_{IO_2} 1.0, peak AwP less than 30 mbar, PEEP 5 to 8 mbar, and f 12 to 16/min. Ventilation is aimed at normocapnia; V_ts should not exceed 6 to 8 mL/kg to avoid pulmonary damage.

Δ Do not start OLV unless airway position is reconfirmed by FOB

Sleeve pneumonectomy and anastomosis Before transection of the trachea, a recruitment maneuver is performed in the ventilated lung. Again, HFJV or CFI-V are used (**Figs. 12** and **13**).

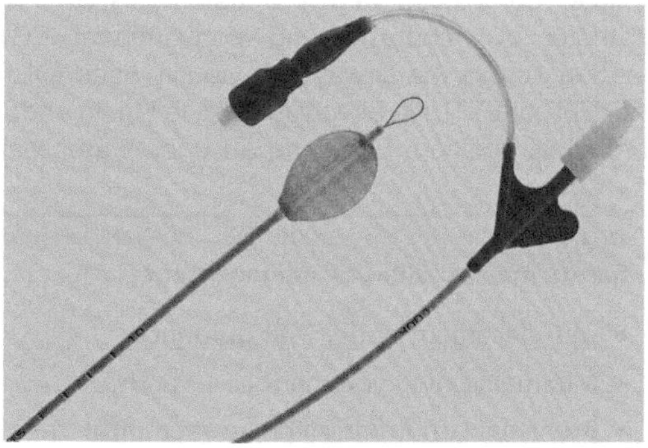

Fig. 10. BB for OLV: Arndt BB catheter featuring a nylon guide loop for blocker placement under FOB guidance. Permission for use granted by Cook Medical Incorporated, Bloomington, Indiana.

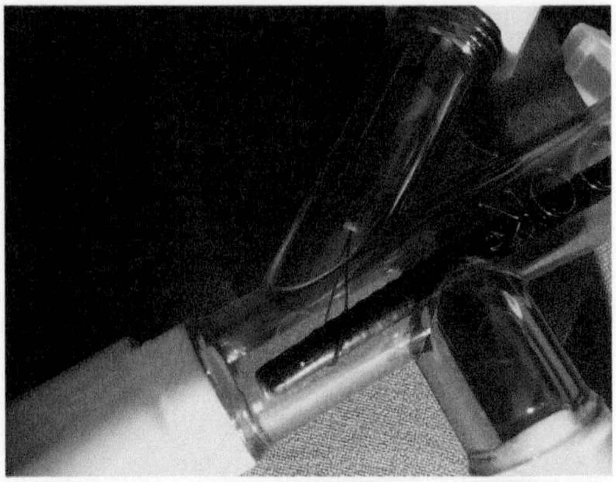

Fig. 11. BB for OLV: multiport airway adapter with blocker port, FOB port, and port to anesthesia circuit. The FOB is engaged by the nylon loop at the tip of the blocker catheter for directing the BB into the target bronchus.

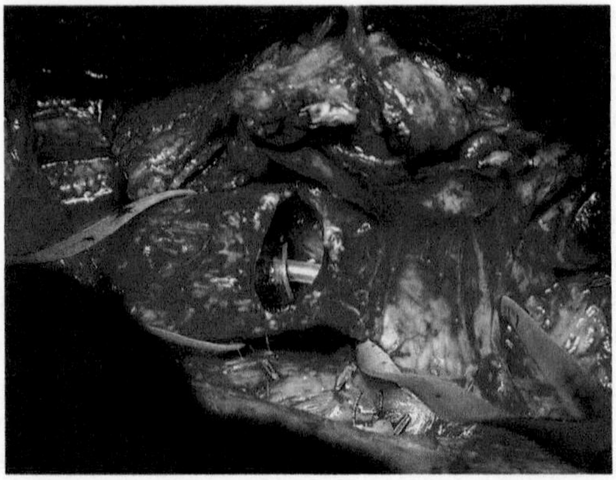

Fig. 12. Jet ventilation during sleeve pneumonectomy. Dorsal aspect of the carinal region with the trachea severed. The DLT used during OLV has been retracted cephalad. Across its bronchial lumen (*blue*) an HFJV catheter has been introduced into the left main bronchus. (*Courtesy of* H. Hoffmann, MD, Thoraxklinik, Heidelberg, Germany.)

a. The DLT is retracted with the tip of the bronchial lumen just above the planned anastomosis (see **Figs. 12** and **13**). On transection, a jet catheter is advanced into the left main bronchus with its tip maintained above the interlobar bifurcation. Management and limitations of HFJV see section HFJV: settings and handling in the page 19.
b. The endobronchial WRETT, having been retracted cephalad before transection of trachea and left main bronchus, is redirected by the surgeon into the open stump for ventilation.
c. The BB is removed after the recruitment maneuver. During sleeve resection, the ETT now serves as a conduit for a jet catheter and HFJV to the left lung.

CFI-V is instituted by intubation of the residual left main bronchus across the surgical field, when during HFJV Pa_{O_2} is less than 60 mm Hg and hypercapnia induces a respiratory acidosis with pH less than 7.1.

After completion of the anastomosis, the jet catheter is withdrawn and conventional PCV started across the airways previously used (DLT, WRETT, or ETT). No airway may be left in an endobronchial position. Following an underwater leak test the anastomosis is inspected by FOB and the bronchial tree cleared of secretions. Airway management and ventilation techniques for carinal resection follow the same pattern.

Box 2
Safety measures in DLT management

- DLT placement under FOB guidance
- Minimal sealing volume for DLT cuffs
- Bronchial cuff inflation postponed until after positioning the patient
- Bronchial cuff pressure monitored continuously

Alternatives for gas exchange during TBS are AO (see section Apneic Oxygenation) or extracorporeal oxygenation (see section Extracorporeal Gas Exchange in TBS).

For postoperative care, the trachea is extubated at the end of the procedure with normothermia, stable circulation, and normal gas exchange attained. The patients are cared for in the ICU for 2 to 3 days.

Complications of special importance to the anesthetist

Retention of secretions from impaired mucociliary transport or insufficient cough is treated by

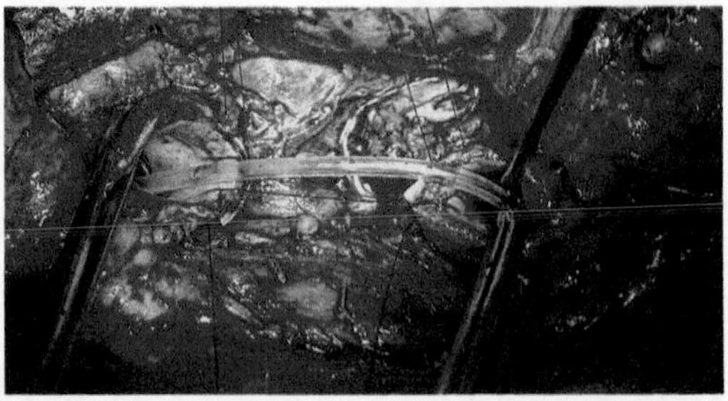

Fig. 13. Jet ventilation during sleeve pneumonectomy. Sleeve pneumonectomy has been completed and placement of sutures commenced. The HFJV catheter is traversing from trachea (*left*) to left main bronchus (*right*). (*Courtesy of* H. Hoffmann, MD, Thoraxklinik, Heidelberg, Germany.)

routine physiotherapy. Liberal use of FOB under local anesthesia for targeted bronchial toilet and inspection of airway anastomoses is preferable to blind nasotracheal suction. Pneumonia is treated by antibiotics according to sensitivity reports. Postpneumonectomy pulmonary edema (PPPE) is a rare differential diagnosis in pneumonia with mortality from 20% to 100%. Because of multifactorial capillary damage and inflammation, PPPE is considered an acute lung injury.[66] Prudent fluid management and lung-protective OLV are preventive.[67] Therapy comprises lung-protective ventilation, pulmonary vasodilators, and extracorporeal lung support. Cardiac herniation is rare. It mostly occurs in the right hemithorax from rupture of pericardiac patch repair after extended pneumonectomy. Rapid circulatory compromise and venous engorgement are key symptoms. As a first step, patients are positioned on their nonsurgical sides. The diagnosis is confirmed by transesophageal echocardiography. Surgical repair is always required. A comprehensive discussion of postoperative complications in TBS is given in the article by Leschber elsewhere in this issue.

Anesthesia and Ventilation for Tracheobronchomalacia

General aspects

Details are discussed in the article by Kugler and Stanzl elsewhere in this issue. Briefly, tracheobronchomalacia (TBM) means loss of structural integrity in tracheal and bronchial cartilages. Dynamic outflow obstruction is the functional consequence of TBM, causing dyspnea, intractable cough, retention of secretions, and recurrent infections.[68] FOB under spontaneous respiration or dynamic computed tomography shows expiratory collapse of the large airways. Posterior tracheoplasty means reapproximation of the tips of the splayed cartilaginous rings in suturing strips of nonabsorbable mesh to the tips as splints bilaterally in the posterior walls of the trachea and main bronchi.[68] During these steps, airway cuffs may get punctured. On completion of tracheobronchoplasty the airways must be inspected by FOB for results requiring corrective steps, such as transmural sutures or airway distortion.

Conduct of anesthesia

General aspects and management of induction in severe cases of TBM are discussed earlier. If FOB under spontaneous ventilation after anesthetic induction is desirable, a supraglottic airway (LMA) provides optimal exposure of TBM.

Management of airways and gas exchange

Posterior splinting tracheoplasty is facilitated by OLV. For separation, 2 types of airways are used:

a. A left-sided DLT is most versatile (see section Management of Airways and Gas Exchange); safety measures to account for the vulnerability of the dilated and distorted tracheobronchial tree must be used (see **Box 2**).
b. The flexibility and small diameter of a WRETT endobronchial tube (see **Fig. 8**) (see section Management of Airways and Gas Exchange) minimize impact on the airways.[25]

Emergence and postoperative phase

The trachea is extubated at the end of the procedure. Because tracheomalacia may extend cranially beyond the tracheoplasty, occasional airway compromise may be encountered. The patients are cared for in the ICU for 2 to 3 days. Mask continuous positive airway pressure may be helpful for internal tracheal splinting (For pain therapy see section on page 17).

SUMMARY

TBS poses challenges to the anesthesiologist. Although the focus is commonly on techniques of gas exchange, conduct of anesthesia and management of airways in the light of the lesions' nature and position in the tracheobronchial tree are equally demanding. Knowledge of procedural requirements, a wide array of techniques for airway management and ventilation, and command of bronchoscopy provide for a consistent plan to merge with surgical intention. Versatile reaction to deviations in anatomy and perioperative course is crucial for safe conduct of delicate surgery on structures vital for gas exchange.

REFERENCES

1. Evans E, Biro P, Bedforth N. Jet ventilation. Cont Educ Anaesth Crit Care Pain 2007;7:2–5.
2. Carlon GC, Cole R, Miodownik S, et al. Physiologic implications of high frequency jet ventilation techniques. Crit Care Med 1983;11:508–14.
3. Young JD, Sykes MK. A method for measuring tidal volume during high frequency jet ventilation. Br J Anaesth 1988;61:601–5.
4. Buczkowski PW, Fombon FN, Lin ES, et al. Air entrainment during high-frequency jet ventilation in a model of upper tracheal stenosis. Br J Anaesth 2007;99:891–7.
5. Bourgain JL, Desruennes E, Cosset MF, et al. Measurement of end-expiratory pressure during transtracheal high frequency jet ventilation for laryngoscopy. Br J Anaesth 1990;65:737–43.

6. Klain M, Smith RB. Fluidic technology. A discussion and a description of a fluidic controlled ventilator for use with high flow oxygen techniques. Anaesthesia 1976;31:750–7.
7. Biro P. Jet ventilation for surgical interventions in the upper airway. Anesthesiol Clin 2010;28:397–409.
8. Cook TM, Alexander R. Major complications during anaesthesia for elective laryngeal surgery in the UK: a national survey of the use of high-pressure source ventilation. Br J Anaesth 2008;101:266–72.
9. Jacquet Y, Monnier P, Van Melle G, et al. Complications of different ventilation strategies in endoscopic laryngeal surgery. A 10-year review. Anesthesiology 2006;104:52–9.
10. Regnard JF, Perrotin C, Giovannnetti R, et al. Resection for tumors with carinal involvement: technical aspects, results, and prognostic factors. Ann Thorac Surg 2005;80:1841–6.
11. Rea F, Marulli G, Schiavon M, et al. Tracheal sleeve pneumonectomy for non small cell lung cancer (NSCLC): short and long-term results in a single institution. Lung Cancer 2008;61:202–8.
12. Zander R, Mertzlufft F. Clinical use of oxygen stores: preoxygenation and apneic oxygenation. In: Erdmann W, Bruley DF, editors. Oxygen transport to tissues XIV. New York: Plenum Press. Adv Exp Med Biol 1992;317:413–20.
13. Biedler A, Mertzlufft F, Feifel G. Apnoeic oxygenation and Boerhaave's syndrome. [Apnoische Oxygenierung bei Boerhaave-Syndrom]. Anasthesiol Intensivmed Notfallmed Schmerzther 1995;30: 257–60 [in German].
14. Nunn JF. Carbon dioxide. In: Nunn JF, editor. Nunn's applied respiratory physiology. Oxford (United Kingdom): Butterworth-Heinemann; 1993. p. 219–46.
15. Rudlof B, Faldum A, Brandt L. Aventilatory mass flow during apnea. Investigations on quantification. [Aventilatorischer Massenfluss während Apnoe. Untersuchungen zur Quantifizierung]. Anaesthesist 2010;59:401–9 [in German].
16. Mertzlufft FO, Brandt L, Stanton-Hicks M, et al. Arterial and mixed venous blood gas status during apnoea of intubation-proof of the Christiansen-Douglas-Haldane effect in vivo. Anaesth Intensive Care 1989;17:325–31.
17. Stock MC, Schisler JQ, McSweeney TD. The $PaCO_2$ rate of rise in anesthetized patients with airway obstruction. J Clin Anesth 1989;1:328–32.
18. Fraioli RL, Sheffer LA, Steffenson JL. Pulmonary and cardiovascular effects of apneic oxygenation in man. Anesthesiology 1973;39:588–96.
19. Frumin J, Epstein RM, Cohen G. Apneic oxygenation in man. Anesthesiology 1959;20:789–98.
20. Holmdahl MH, Wiklund L, Wetterberg T, et al. The place of THAM in the management of acidemia in clinical practice. Acta Anaesthesiol Scand 2000; 44:524–7.
21. Höstman SH, Engström J, Hedenstierna G, et al. Intensive buffering can keep pH above 7.2 for over 4 h during apnea: an experimental porcine study. Acta Anaesthesiol Scand 2013;57:63–70.
22. Nunn JF. The effects of changes in the carbon dioxide tension. In: Nunn JF, editor. Nunn's applied respiratory physiology. Oxford (United Kingdom): Butterworth-Heinemann; 1993. p. 518–28.
23. Pollock JM, Deibler AR, Whitlow CT, et al. Hypercapnia-induced cerebral hyperperfusion, an underrecognized clinical entity. AJNR Am J Neuroradiol 2009;30:378–85.
24. Macchiarini P, Altmayer M, Go T, et al. Technical innovations of carinal resection for nonsmall-cell lung cancer. Ann Thorac Surg 2006;82:1989–97.
25. Wilkey BJ, Alfille P, Weitzel NS, et al. Anesthesia for tracheobronchial surgery. Semin Cardiothorac Vasc Anesth 2012;16:209–19.
26. Jungebluth P, Alici E, Baiguera S, et al. Tracheobronchial transplantation with a stem-cell-seeded bioartificial nanocomposite: a proof-of-concept study. Lancet 2011;378:1997–2004.
27. Jimenez MJ, Sadurni M, Tio M, et al. Apnoeic oxygenation in complex tracheal surgery. Eur J Anaesthesiol 2006;23(Suppl 38):20 Abstract 58.
28. Jense HG, Dubin SA, Silverstein PI, et al. Effect of obesity on safe duration of apnea in anesthetized humans. Anesth Analg 1991;72:89–93.
29. Macchiarini P, Rovira I, Ferrarello S. Awake upper airway surgery. Ann Thorac Surg 2010;89:387–91.
30. Bonnet F, Derosier JP, Pluskwa F, et al. Cervical epidural anaesthesia for carotid artery surgery. Can J Anaesth 1990;37:353–8.
31. Baylot D, Mahul P, Navez ML, et al. Cervical epidural anaesthesia. [Anesthésie péridurale cervicale]. Ann Fr Anesth Reanim 1993;12:483–92 [in French].
32. Hakl M, Michalek P, Sevcik P, et al. Regional anaesthesia for carotid endarterectomy: an audit over 10 years. Br J Anaesth 2007;99:415–20.
33. Dohi S, Nishikawa T, Ujike Y, et al. Circulatory responses to airway stimulation and cervical epidural blockade. Anesthesiology 1982;57:359–63.
34. Takasaki M, Takahashi T. Respiratory function during cervical and thoracic extradural analgesia in patients with normal lungs. Br J Anaesth 1980;52: 1271–6.
35. Capdevila X, Biboulet P, Rubenovitch J, et al. The effects of cervical epidural anesthesia with bupivacaine on pulmonary function in conscious patients. Anesth Analg 1998;86:1033–8.
36. Giebler RM, Scherer RU, Peters J. Incidence of neurologic complications related to thoracic epidural catheterization. Anesthesiology 1997;86: 55–63.
37. Pöpping DM, Zahn PK, Van Aken HK, et al. Effectiveness and safety of postoperative pain

management: a survey of 18 925 consecutive patients between 1998 and 2006 (2nd revision): a database analysis of prospectively raised data. Br J Anaesth 2008;101:832–40.
38. Wiebe K, Baraki H, Macchiarini P, et al. Extended pulmonary resections of advanced thoracic malignancies with support of cardiopulmonary bypass. Eur J Cardiothorac Surg 2006;29:571–8.
39. Lang G, Taghavi S, Aigner C, et al. Extracorporeal membrane oxygenation support for resection of locally advanced thoracic tumors. Ann Thorac Surg 2011;92:264–71.
40. Chiu CL, The BT, Wang CY. Temporary cardiopulmonary bypass and isolated lung ventilation for tracheal stenosis and reconstruction. Br J Anaesth 2003;91:742–4.
41. Fromes Y, Gaillard D, Ponzio O, et al. Reduction of the inflammatory response following coronary bypass grafting with total minimal extracorporeal circulation. Eur J Cardiothorac Surg 2002;22:527–33.
42. Müller T, Bein T, Philipp A, et al. Extracorporeal pulmonary support in severe pulmonary failure in adults. Dtsch Arztebl Int 2013;110:159–66.
43. Ius F, Kuehn C, Tudorache I, et al. Lung transplantation on cardiopulmonary support: venoarterial extracorporeal membrane oxygenation outperformed cardiopulmonary bypass. J Thorac Cardiovasc Surg 2012;144:1510–6.
44. Sanchez-Lorente D, Iglesias M, Rodriguez A, et al. The pumpless extracorporeal lung membrane provides complete respiratory support during complex airway reconstructions without inducing cellular trauma or a coagulatory and inflammatory response. J Thorac Cardiovasc Surg 2012;144:425–30.
45. Korvenoja P, Pitkänen O, Berg E, et al. Venovenous extracorporeal membrane oxygenation in surgery for bronchial repair. Ann Thorac Surg 2008;86:1348–9.
46. Kim JE, Jung SH, Ma DS. Experiences of tracheal procedure assisted by extracorporeal membrane oxygenator. Korean J Thorac Cardiovasc Surg 2013;46:80–3.
47. Müller T, Lubnow M, Philipp A, et al. Extracorporeal pumpless interventional lung assist in clinical practice: determinants of efficacy. Eur Respir J 2009;33: 551–8.
48. Wiebe K, Poeling J, Arlt M, et al. Thoracic surgical procedures supported by a pumpless interventional lung assist. Ann Thorac Surg 2010;89: 1782–8.
49. Walles T, Steger V, Wurst H, et al. Pumpless extracorporeal gas exchange aiding central airway surgery. J Thorac Cardiovasc Surg 2008;136:1372–4.
50. Colt HG, Harrell JH. Therapeutic rigid bronchoscopy allows level of care changes in patients with acute respiratory failure from central airways obstruction. Chest 1997;112:202–6.
51. Ramsay MA, Saha D, Hebeler RF. Tracheal resection in the morbidly obese patient: the role of dexmedetomidine. J Clin Anesth 2006;18:452–4.
52. Abdelmalak B, Makary L, Hoban J, et al. Dexmedetomidine as sole sedative for awake intubation in management of the critical airway. J Clin Anesth 2007;19:370–3.
53. Abdelmalak B, Marcanthony N, Abdelmalak J, et al. Dexmedetomidine for anesthetic management of anterior mediastinal mass. J Anesth 2010;24:607–10.
54. Purugganan RV. Intravenous anesthesia for thoracic procedures. Curr Opin Anaesthesiol 2008;21:1–7.
55. Nouraei SA, Giussani DA, Howard DJ, et al. Physiological comparison of spontaneous and positive-pressure ventilation in laryngotracheal stenosis. Br J Anaesth 2008;101:419–23.
56. Hobai IA, Chhangani SV, Alfille PH. Anesthesia for tracheal resection and reconstruction. Anesthesiol Clin 2012;30:709–30.
57. Powell ES, Cook D, Pearce AC, et al. A prospective, multicentre, observational cohort study of analgesia and outcome after pneumonectomy. Br J Anaesth 2011;106:364–70.
58. Brull SJ, Murphy GS. Residual neuromuscular block: lessons unlearned. Part II: methods to reduce the risk of residual weakness. Anesth Analg 2010;111:129–40.
59. Torossian A. Thermal management during anesthesia and thermoregulation standards for the prevention of inadvertent perioperative hypothermia. Best Pract Res Clin Anaesthesiol 2008;22:659–68.
60. Lorenz RR. Adult laryngotracheal stenosis: etiology and surgical management. Curr Opin Otolaryngol Head Neck Surg 2003;11:467–72.
61. Adelsmayr E, Keller C, Erd G, et al. The laryngeal mask and high frequency jet ventilation for resection of high tracheal stenosis. Anesth Analg 1998;86:907–8.
62. Biro P, Hegi TR, Weder W, et al. Laryngeal mask airway and high-frequency jet ventilation for the resection of a high-grade upper tracheal stenosis. J Clin Anesth 2001;13:141–3.
63. Malik MA, Subramaniam R, Maharaj CH, et al. Randomized controlled trial of the Pentax AWS, Glidescope and Macintosh laryngoscopes in predicted difficult intubation. Br J Anaesth 2009;103:761–8.
64. Grillo HC. Reconstruction of the trachea. Experience in 100 consecutive cases. Thorax 1973;28:667–79.
65. Şentürk M. New concepts of the management of one-lung ventilation. Curr Opin Anaesthesiol 2006;19:1–4.
66. Gothard J. Lung injury after thoracic surgery and one-lung ventilation. Curr Opin Anaesthesiol 2006;19:5–10.
67. Della Rocca G, Coccia C. Acute lung injury in thoracic surgery. Curr Opin Anaesthesiol 2013;26:40–6.
68. Damle SS, Mitchell JD. Surgery for tracheobronchomalacia. Semin. Cardiothorac Vasc Anesth 2012;16: 203–8.

Endoscopic Treatment of Tracheal Stenosis

Lutz Freitag*, Kaid Darwiche

KEYWORDS

• Tracheal stenosis • Tracheal tumor • Tracheal stricture • Interventional pneumology
• Laser resection • Airway stent

KEY POINTS

- For tracheal stenoses, surgery with sleeve resection remains the gold standard.
- Interventional techniques through bronchoscopes including laser or electro resection, balloon dilatation and stent placement provide immediate relief from dyspnea.
- Stent placement for benign stenoses and malacias should only be considered if all other options are exhausted because side-effects can hardly be avoided.
- Migration, retained secretions and granulation tissue development are common complications. Newer stents from smarter materials may solve some of the problems.
- Tracheal obstructions require a multidisciplinary approach. Interventional pulmonologists, ENT- and thoracic surgeons must combine their efforts and techniques for the benefit of the patient.

Tracheal stenosis is a debilitating, potentially life-threatening disorder. It can be grouped into categories according to the underlying disease (malignant or benign), the biomechanical properties (scarring strictures or collapsing malacic segments), the functional behavior (fixed or functional), the degree and extension (narrowing, long, or short), or treatment options (operable or inoperable). For patients, it is usually irrelevant what causes their stenoses. They have the same symptoms: stridor, shortness of breath increasing under exercise, and inability to clear secretions because of an impaired cough function. There is no universal classification. With several leading centers in Europe and the United States, we have proposed a classification system.[1] The chart that has been agreed on has proved helpful for describing and grading most central airway stenoses. This article groups the tracheal stenoses mainly according to the endoscopic treatment options. However, an initial distinction between malignant and benign stenoses is practical.

MALIGNANT STENOSES

Malignant tumors of the lung, the esophagus, the thyroid, or other mediastinal structures often involve the trachea by direct tumor growth, invasion, or lymph node compression. Primary tracheal cancers are less common than other types of lung cancer. They can be found at any age because they are not always related to a smoking history. Our youngest patient with a primary inoperable squamous cell cancer that had developed from a tracheostomy scar was 15 years old.[2] The youngest patient with a tracheal scar carcinoma in the literature was 6 years old. We have seen another 15-year-old boy with an inoperable adenoid cystic carcinoma. Both were short of breath when we performed bronchoscopy. One reason why these children were already inoperable when finally diagnosed is the years of misdiagnoses of childhood asthma. At the other end of the spectrum, we found a huge small cell cancer obstructing the trachea of a 70-year-old patient with chronic obstructive

The authors have nothing to disclose.
Department of Interventional Pulmonology, Ruhrlandklinik, University Hospital, University Duisburg-Essen, 45239 Essen, Germany
* Corresponding author.
E-mail address: lutz.freitag@ruhrlandklinik.uk-essen.de

Thorac Surg Clin 24 (2014) 27–40
http://dx.doi.org/10.1016/j.thorsurg.2013.10.003
1547-4127/14/$ – see front matter

pulmonary disease who could not be weaned in a weaning center.[3] The message is clear but should be repeated again: unclear dyspnea is an indication for bronchoscopy.

Although clinical symptoms and pulmonary function test determine the urge of bronchoscopy, imaging methods help in planning the procedure. Computed tomography or magnetic resonance imaging can guide the preparation of instruments. If images show an obstruction from intraluminal tumor growth (**Fig. 1**A) a cutting device such as an electrical snare should be prepared. The compression from extrinsic tumor growth in the other patient (see **Fig. 1**B) indicated that he might need a stent. In cases of severe central airway obstruction, whether they are malignant or nonmalignant, it is important to stabilize the patient first and then make interdisciplinary treatment decisions.[4]

OBSTRUCTING MALIGNANT TUMORS

As soon as a tracheal tumor is revealed by bronchoscopy, a rapid decision has to be made whether immediate treatment is required or not. Passing an almost obstructing tumor with a flexible bronchoscope, especially if combined with taking a biopsy, can cause a life-threatening situation because of swelling or bleeding. In contrast, an unreflected laser resection or a hasty stent insertion can jeopardize a potential curative operation. Using a rigid bronchoscope and a coagulation device that enables maintenance of airway patency is safer. Whatever bronchoscopists do to diagnose and treat, they should always consider contacting a surgeon. Despite all the available tools, sleeve resection may be the only curative option. It is a good idea to take biopsies first from potential resection spots, before the tumor is touched with a forceps. Autofluorescence bronchoscopy can help to identify tumor margins.

The best-established instrument for destroying intraluminally growing tumors is the laser. Neodymium yttrium aluminum garnet (ND-YAG) or infrared diode lasers guide the photoenergy through flexible glass fibers that are easily passed through the working channel of a bronchoscope. It is a never-ending debate whether such a procedure can be done safely enough with a flexible bronchoscope or whether rigid instruments are required. For malignant tracheal tumors, we prefer to intubate the patient with a rigid bronchoscope under general anesthesia and jet ventilation and insert a flexible videochip bronchoscopy through the open rigid endoscope. We are convinced that this is the safest approach, proving best airway control. When dealing with very high tracheal tumors, we opt for a Kleinsasser laryngoscope with a jet ventilation nozzle. Teamwork with anesthesiologists and assistance is mandatory. Before using a laser, we make sure that the patient is ventilated with a gas mixture of not more than 40% oxygen. A typical laser is set to energy levels between 15 and 25 W for coagulation and 25 to 40 W for resection. With a distance of 5 to 10 mm between the tip of the fiber and the tumor surface, photocoagulation and resection is performed with short pulses of 0.5 seconds (**Fig. 2**).

Laser resection is safe if guidelines are followed.[5] Dumon and colleagues[6] reported a mortality of 1 in 1000 benign and 5 in 1000 malignant cases in a series of almost 5100 patients. One risk that has to be kept in mind is a potential ignition hazard if the hot laser beam reaches inflammable objects such as endotracheal cannulas or stents. Although most reports and studies are of the original ND-YAG laser, there are now smaller and less expensive diode lasers that can be shared among departments because they are transportable and do not require water cooling. However, even these new devices are not cheap and clinicians look for feasible alternative instruments. The original coring-out technique with the tip of a rigid bronchoscope is still the fastest technique. However, bleeding and perforation are dangers and most clinicians prefer to have a coagulating device at hand. Any surgical electrocautery device can be used for the removal of

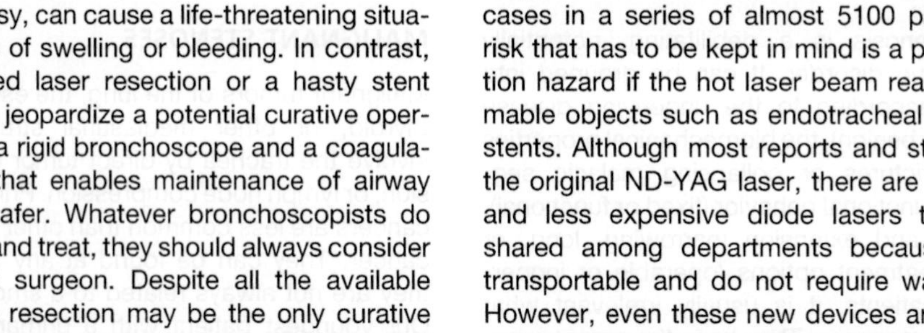

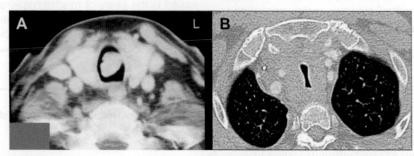

Fig. 1. Intraluminal tumor growth (*A*) can be treated with endoscopic cutting devices. Extrinsic compression is probably treated best with stent insertion (*B*).

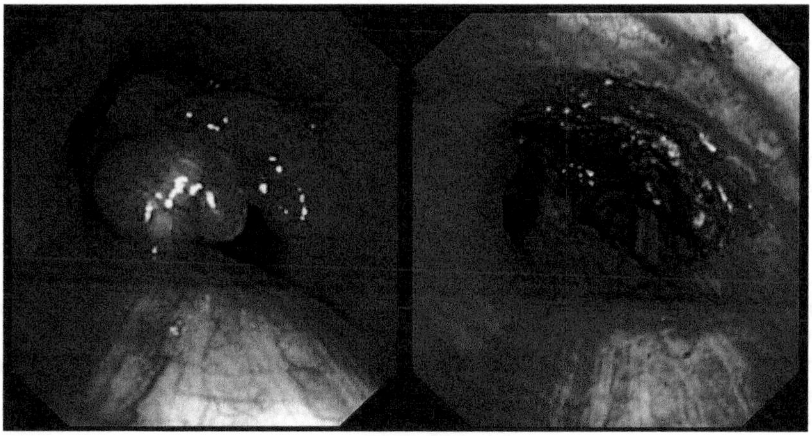

Fig. 2. A malignant tracheal tumor is photoresected with an ND-YAG laser.

obstructing tracheal tumors, provided that feasible probes and insulated bronchoscopes are used.[7] Less expensive but more common are argon plasma coagulation (APC) devices. Instead of a metal contact probe, ionized argon gas transports the energy to the tumor surface and vessels.[8] In contrast with a laser beam that always delivers the energy straight forward, the direction of the argon gas beam is influenced by the electrical conductivity of the tissue. Therefore, vessel-rich tumors or bleeding lesions are preferentially reached and coagulated. Because aiming is not as precise as the laser, and vessels in the vicinity of a tumor are also coagulated because of the mechanism mentioned earlier, caution is required not to damage unaffected tissue if surgery (sleeve resection) is still considered. The depth of penetration is lower than with an infrared laser and removal procedures take longer (**Fig. 3**).

The risk of ignition is almost negligible because the argon gas flushes the oxygen away. However, there is a device-related risk. If the argon gas fiber accidentally reaches into a vascularized tumor, argon gas can penetrate into the tissue vessels, potentially resulting in coronary or brain gas embolisms.[9] As a precaution, a distance of 5 mm between the argon beam and the tumor should be maintained, as with a laser fiber.

The third instrument that can accomplish tumor removal from central airway is the cryoprobe.[10,11] Using the Joule-Thomson effect, a gas conducted from a tank through a catheter rapidly expands, causing extreme cold at the metal tip that is pressed against the tumor. There are bigger semirigid probes that require a rigid bronchoscope, but smaller catheters that can be inserted through the working channel of a flexible bronchoscope are equally feasible. There are 2 techniques based on different modes of action. The cryoprobe can be used to freeze a tumor and turn it into an ice block. Pulling out the still-cold catheter rips out this frozen tumor block. Cryorecanalization is not

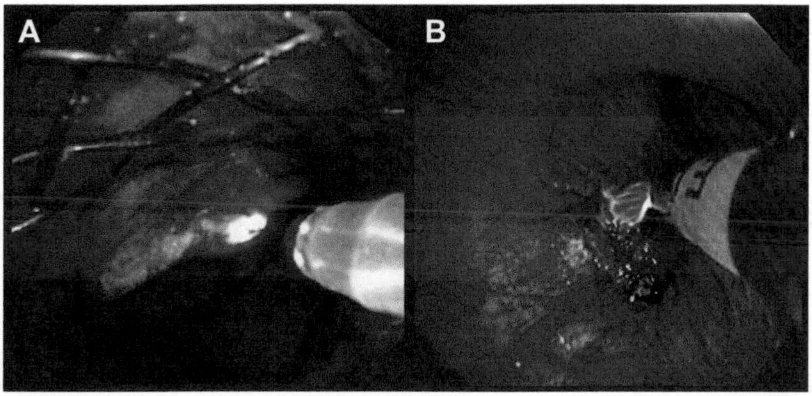

Fig. 3. The laser beam (*A*) goes straight forward, making cutting precise but coagulation sometimes difficult. The argon gas beam (*B*) follows the best electrical conductivity. APC is a less precise cutting instrument but an almost ideal coagulation device.

a blood-free procedure. However, it has some advantages besides its speed of action. Cartilages are more cold resistant than other airway structures. Thus the cryoextraction has a selective effect. It is advantageous to combine it with coagulation technique such as APC. The clinical nickname of this combination technique is fire and ice. We use it more for the removal of excessive granulation tissue than for the removal of malignant tumors. Cryorecanalization is another fast physical removal procedure with efficiencies and risks comparable with laser or electrocautery. A cryodevice can also be used for a biologic technique that is usually referred to as classic cryotherapy. Several cycles of freezing and thawing are applied to a tumor without ripping it off. These freeze-thawing cycles induce apoptosis or necrosis with an even more selective effect on malignant tumors. However, this destructive effect on tumor tissue is retarded. It can take several days until the treated tissue dies. Because it does not provide immediate tumor shrinkage, classic cryotherapy it is not a feasible option for patients with severely obstructing tumors.

Another treatment modality for intratracheal cancers is photodynamic therapy, which is a complex multistep approach. First, a sensitizing drug is given intravenously. The drug accumulates to some degree inside tumor tissue. Most drugs, such as the porphyrines, have fluorescent properties. When illuminated with blue-violet light, they emit bright red light. This effect has been used to detect small cancers. For treatment, the drug-rich tumor is illuminated with red light from a laser source. This light induces the photodynamic process with a release of singlet oxygen causing vessel shutdown and apoptosis in the tumor tissue. Tumor cells are destroyed as selectively as possible. Older drugs, such as the approved Photofrin, cause skin sensitivity. Patients can develop sunburn when exposed to normal daylight. Patients had to stay in darkened rooms for several days or even weeks. However, newer sensitizers have shorter half-lives. The photosensitivity of chlorins that we are currently using in studies limits the out-of-light phase to a single day. Photodynamic therapy for obstructing tracheal tumors is a complex and expansive procedure but it is often the best chance for patients who are inoperable (**Fig. 4**).[12]

Another option that is not common but might have great potential is the intratumoral injection of chemotherapy drugs with a needle through the working channel of a bronchoscope.[13,14]

NONOBSTRUCTING INTRALUMINAL TUMORS

At early stages tracheal tumors do not cause symptoms. These nonobstructing primary tracheal tumors should not be classified as stage T4 lung tumors; the designation of T1 is used for superficial tumors limited to the airway wall. They are considered operable unless they have metastasized or technical problems or patient comorbidities exclude surgery. For the time being, surgery remains the gold standard of therapy. The most common alternative for inoperable tracheal cancer is radiation therapy, usually combined with a platinum-based chemotherapy. However, if there are smaller lesions, endoscopic therapy may be used with curative intent. The success rate depends on the extension and the invasion depth of the tumor. Fluorescence bronchoscopy and endobronchial ultrasound help in selecting the optimal treatment modality. If the tumor is not longer than 2 cm and respects the tracheal wall, the bronchoscopic techniques mentioned earlier can reach local tumor eradication rates of up to 80%. For recurrent cancers and cancers that

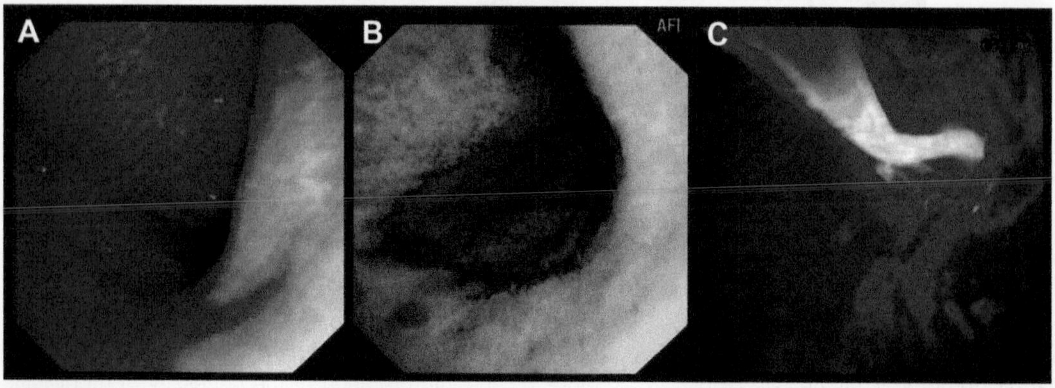

Fig. 4. Early cancers are hardly visible with white light bronchoscopy (*A*). Autofluorescence bronchoscopy helps to detect and delineate such tumors (*B*). Photodynamic therapy with red light is applied to treat the low-volume tumor growing in the lower third of the trachea (*C*).

extend through the tracheal wall, high-dose-rate brachytherapy may be offered as a potentially curative measure. Brachytherapy requires good cooperation between the endoscopist and the radiation oncologist. Because it is technically less demanding, some centers prefer external stereotactic radiation therapy rather than endotracheal brachytherapy, with the drawback of increased radiation dose in lung tissue. Many bronchoscopy-based antineoplastic therapies complement each other and their effects are additive. In selected cases, we have combined laser resection, classic cryotherapy, and brachytherapy or photodynamic therapy and brachytherapy (**Fig. 5**).[12]

EXTRINSIC TUMOR COMPRESSION AND WALL DESTRUCTION

Although lasers, cautery devices, or cryoprobes are most helpful for removing intraluminal cancers, they are useless for treating submucosal or extrabronchial lesions. If lymph nodes or other tumors compress the trachea from outside or if the wall is already destroyed, none of the cutting or coagulation devices is applicable. These conditions require splinting with an airway stent. We hardly ever find pure extrinsic compression with unaffected airway walls. If cancer grows inside as well as outside of the central airways, endoscopic treatment techniques may be combined. Most often, intraluminally growing tumor tissue is first removed with a laser or APC and then a stent is inserted to stabilize the effect. We prefer to perform these interventions with rigid bronchoscopy under general anesthesia, as explained before. Combining coagulation, mechanical debulking, and stent insertion provides immediate and long-lasting relief from dyspnea (**Fig. 6**).

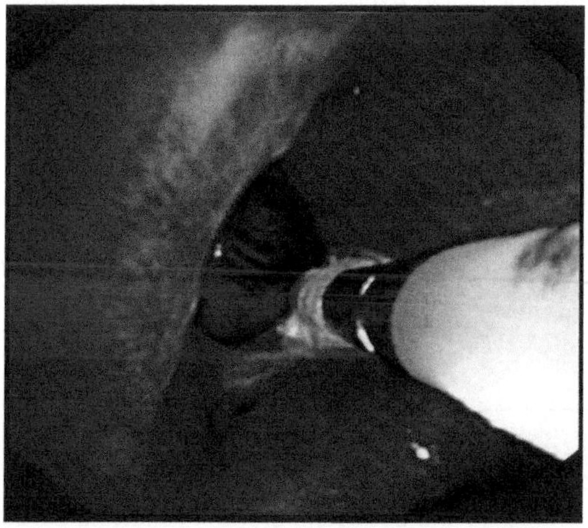

Fig. 5. Classic cryotherapy is used with curative intent to destroy a small early tracheal cancer.

With a stent in place, the patient can receive chemotherapy or radiation therapy. If these tumor-destructive treatments are successful, the stent may be removed a few weeks later. This approach does not prohibit surgery if a potentially removable stent has been used. A plethora of airway stents is commercially available.[15,16] They all have advantages and disadvantages. Silicone stents must be inserted through rigid bronchoscopes, but self-expanding metal stents can be implanted with flexible instruments. Silicone stents are easier to reposition or to remove. For the treatment of malignant stenoses, we only recommend silicone stents or fully covered metal stents. If an uncovered stent has become embedded in the tissue it cannot be removed without severe harm to the mucosa. Tumor tissue can easily grow through the meshes of uncovered stents. If the carinal region is involved, bifurcated stents are preferable. All currently available bifurcated stents can be removed bronchoscopically by grabbing their upper ends with a forceps and pulling them out through the larynx under the protection of a rigid bronchoscope. The Dynamic stent has incorporated steel clasps and others are made from nitinol. With little metal mass, the Y-shaped stents do not interfere with radiation therapy (**Fig. 7**).[17]

BENIGN TRACHEAL TUMORS

For the treatment of semimalignant or benign tumors growing inside the trachea, any of the removal techniques mentioned earlier can be applied. Whether a patient is operable or not depends on the extent of the tumor. In several cases, we have first used laser resection as an immediate measure and have later performed surgical sleeve resection. Everybody has a favorite technique. For the removal of fibroadenomas, we have successfully used the electrical snare. Amyloid tumors can be treated with laser, followed by external beam radiation or brachytherapy. Cryotherapy is particularly safe for the treatment of papillomatosis. These tumors also respond well to photodynamic therapy, although none of the available drugs has been approved for this indication.

BENIGN TRACHEAL STRICTURES

There are many different entities and types of benign tracheal stenoses. Following a physical or chemical irritation (eg, from a tracheal tube), an inflammatory cascade is started. Transforming growth factor beta upregulation promotes the growth of fibroblast, which are less demanding than epithelial cells.[18] A disturbed healing process causes an imbalance of cells types, with scarring

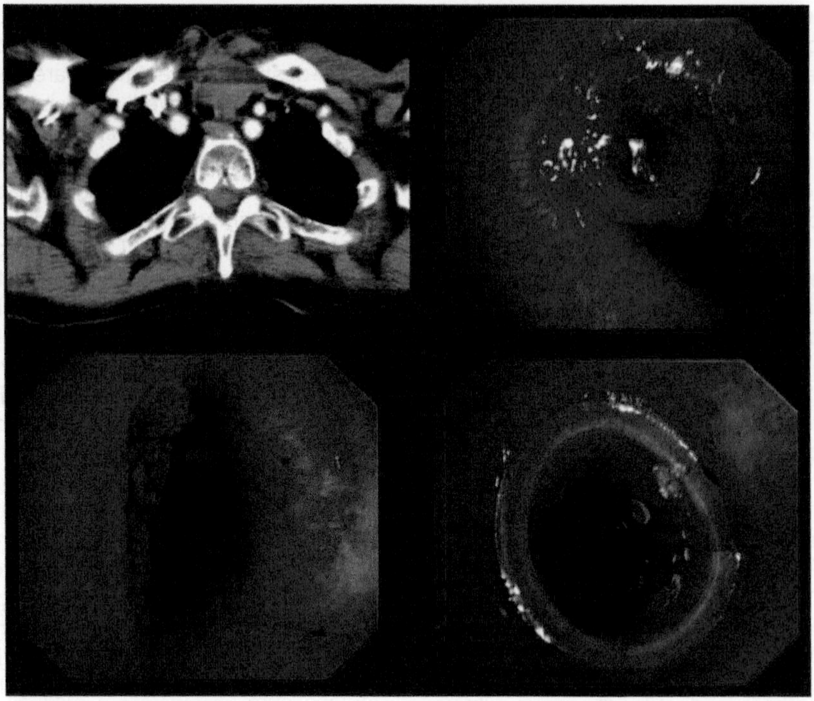

Fig. 6. A tracheal cancer with extrinsic and intraluminal components severely impairs tracheal airflow. Following laser resection of the intratracheal tumor portion, a Dumon silicone stent is placed to stabilize the effect.

and excessive growth of granulation tissue. Fibroblasts release collagen and an extracellular matrix replaces the normal healthy and patent airway. With less elastin and more collagen, stenoses become rigid and cannot be passed with flexible instruments. The most serious mucosal damage we have seen was in patients who had inhaled mustard gas.[19] However, any injury, whether physical or chemical, can result in severe airway narrowing. In most cases, excessive granulation tissue formation, sometimes in types of polyps, deteriorates the situation. The damage is not usually limited to the mucosa but reaches deep into cartilage structures. The normal biomechanical function of the horseshoe-shaped tracheal cartilages is to create tension to keep the trachea patent. If the cartilages are destroyed, weakened, or fractured, the trachea collapses during rapid exhalation and coughing. Most clinicians call this disturbance true malacia, distinguishing it from the other type of airway collapse. If the posterior wall bulges inward, sometimes to a degree that posterior and anterior walls touch during coughing, it is called excessive central airway collapse.

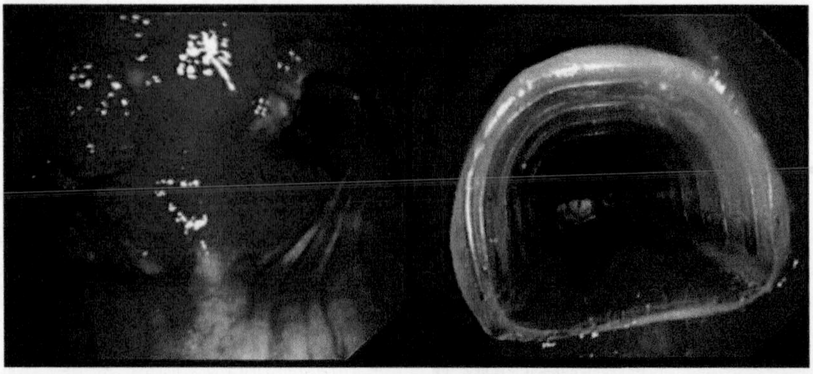

Fig. 7. A malignant tumor involving the carinal region with trachea and both stem bronchi. Following partial removal of cancer tissue with a laser, a bifurcated Dynamic stent has been inserted, providing immediate relief of dyspnea.

This type is often seen in patients with emphysema. Pulmonary function tests with forced maneuvers help to distinguish the different entities. Rigid stenoses, including those from granulation tissue, affect inspiratory as well as expiratory peak flow. Collapse syndromes mainly affect the expiratory flow curve, often with an almost normal airway resistance in the shutter technique of body plethysmography. In order to avoid underdiagnosis, forced maneuvers for function tests have to be ordered. We call this the tracheal stenosis program, which includes forced inhalation and expiration maneuvers, sometimes with different head positions.

The main types of benign stenoses are shown in **Fig. 8**. There are short web-type stenoses with scar tissue, hourglass-shaped long stenoses with airway wall thickening, damaged cartilages resulting in saber-sheath malacia, and collapsing segments from unproportional broad and floppy posterior membranes. We often encounter a mixture of malacic and rigid strictures, all contributing to functional tracheal narrowing (**Fig. 9**).

WEB STENOSES

Web stenoses are found in systemic diseases such as Wegener granulomatosis. They often result from a localized trauma or irritation, such as aspiration. An inflammation is followed by growth of rigid scar tissue. A common mistake is a simple dilatation or bouginage. It provides immediate relief but is usually not long lasting; because healthy tissue is weaker and softer, it is ruptured first, whereas the stronger scar tissue is more resistant. These microtraumas to the formerly unaffected mucosa are the initial stimuli for a recurrence. The same effect is seen if a laser with deep coagulation properties is used. Vessels supplying the healthy tissue are shut down and new granulation tissue formation is initiated. For the same reason, circumferential cutting must be avoided because it impairs blood supply and fluid exchange, thereby favoring growth of the less demanding fibroblasts while epithelial cells and cartilages are further damaged.[20] This collateral damage can be avoided if more appropriate techniques are used. Based on these theoretic considerations and clinical experience, we use and recommend a 2-step procedure for the treatment of a short web stenosis. First, we make a few precise cuts into the scar, preferably into the anterior part of the web to make sure that the posterior membrane of the trachea is not damaged. Once small radial cuts have been made, the stenosis can be carefully dilated. Following this pretreatment, the scarred tissue ruptures at the desired spots. Because of the typical appearance of the cuts, it is referred to as the Mickey Mouse ears technique. Even more precise cuts than with a laser can be achieved with an electrosurgical knife.[21] Attached to a standard HF generator, the catheter probe is passed through the working channel of a routine bronchoscope and pressed against the scar. Under direct visualization, scars can be cut and removed with minimal side effects on healthy tissue. There is less fibrin production after electro cutting than after laser therapy. For web insertion, APC is less appropriate because good vascularized healthy tissue is a better electrical conductor than the dry extracellular matrix that is targeted (**Fig. 10**).

STRICTURES

Strictures are different from web-type stenoses. Often resulting from long-term intubation or other physical damage, the tracheal wall is thickened, partially from cells and partially from extracellular matrix, especially collagen. Cartilages are deformed and weakened. The stenosis has an hourglass shape, without an abrupt step. It is difficult to

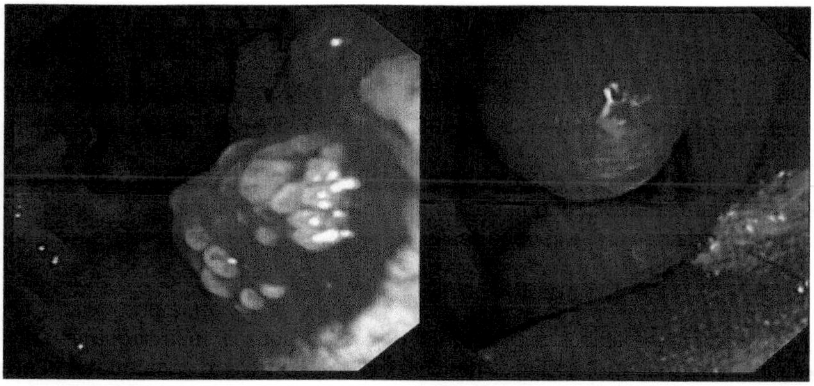

Fig. 8. Benign tumors such as a papillomatosis or fibroadenomas can obstruct a trachea as severely as a malignant tumor.

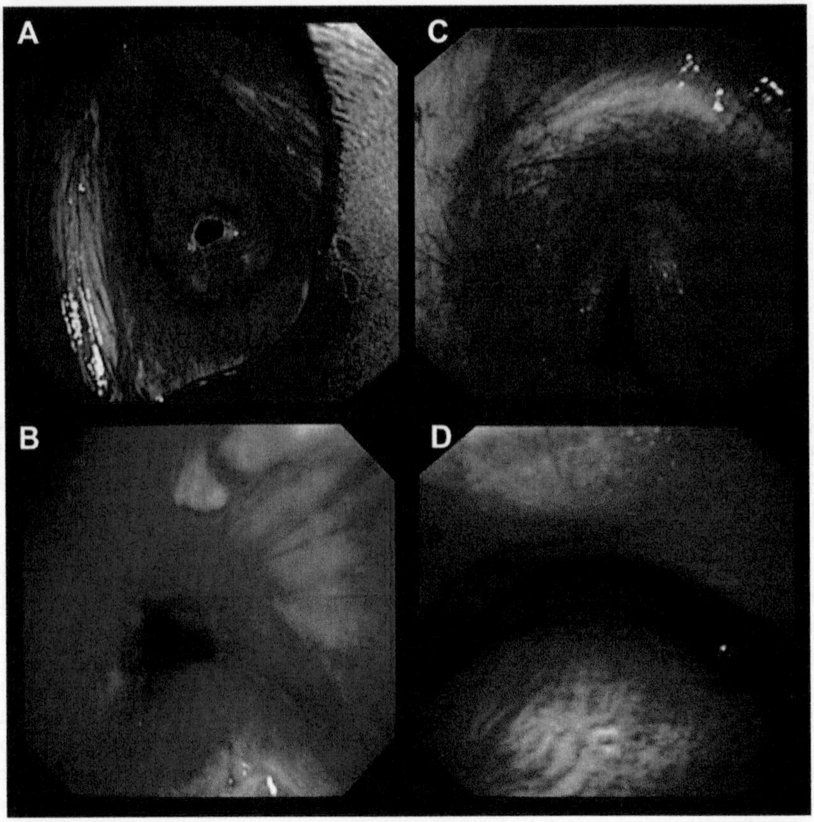

Fig. 9. There are 4 different types of benign tracheal stenoses. (*A*) A short web stenosis, (*B*) a long chronic inflammatory (hourglass) stenosis, (*C*) a postintubation stenosis with damaged cartilages, and (*D*) tracheomalacia.

judge where the stenosis begins and ends if surgery is planned. For a successful outcome of a sleeve resection it is mandatory to anastomose only healthy, unaffected cartilages and mucosa. The extension of the damage often limits respective surgical options. For the time being, because tracheal transplant or other replacements are still experimental, endoscopic techniques remain the treatment standards. They include laser resection of granulation tissue, dilatation, stent placement, or tracheotomy.

DILATATION

Long stenoses that cannot be corrected surgically are treated bronchoscopically. Typical approaches are bouginage or dilatation. Any tapered bronchoscope or a bougie can be used to dilate a stricture.

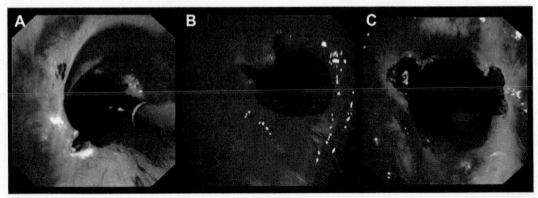

Fig. 10. An electrical knife (*A*) or a laser is used to make radial insertion into the web stenosis. Once the Mickey Mouse ears are cut (*B*), dilation can be performed with less risk of damaging healthy tissue (*C*).

Some clinicians prefer using a balloon. From a physical perspective, the main difference between the techniques is the vector of the force. Pushing wedge instruments forward applies force at an angle, whereas a balloon applies force perpendicular. If a soft, highly compliant balloon is used (eg, a latex balloon of a Fogarty catheter) the healthy tissue is overstretched. Therefore, only low-compliance Gruentzig-type balloons similar to those that are supplied for angioplasty purposes should be used. Although balloon dilatation has become popular, its biomechanical effect is poorly understood. If stress (eg, from the pressure in a balloon) is applied to any tissue, strain (deformation) results in a time-dependant manner. Water is squeezed out, collagen is ruptured, and the stenosis opens slowly. The behavior is viscous, meaning it takes some time. The stenosis opens but partially closes again if the stress is released (balloon emptied). This part could be described as elastic. In most cases, the lumen does not shrink back to its initial extent. The area remains wider than before. This plastic deformation is what is needed in a dilation procedure. Although the physics of balloon dilatation have been investigated[22] and clinical results are promising,[23,24] hardly anything is known about the biologic effects. It is not known how long a stenosis should be dilated. The viscous properties of tracheal scars have not been investigated. Because the trachea is completely occluded during the dilatation procedure, the time that the expanding force is applied is limited to less than a minute. It is also not known how much pressure is most appropriate. The reading on the gauge meter does not reflect the constrictive force of a stenosis but only the physical property of a balloon. It might be that a soft dilatation with slightly increasing pressure over several hours would result in better clinical outcomes. However, no instruments are available that could determine the specific stress-strain relationship of an individual tracheal stenosis. For the time being, we use an angioplasty balloon with a nominal diameter of, for example, 14 mm and fill it with diluted contrast medium under the recommended pressure (mostly 6–8 bar) under fluoroscopy. We wait until the waist of the balloon disappears, as shown in **Fig. 11**.

STENTS IN BENIGN STRICTURES

If surgery is not possible and dilatation has only a temporary effect, the next treatment option is stent placement. This option is the most debated procedure. Placing a stent does not require particular skills and the procedure is well reimbursed, which makes it challenging for anyone who owns a bronchoscope and runs a department. Making the clinically correct decision requires more skills than the procedure. We have been dealing with young patients who have had accidents and with people who developed a tracheal stenosis after an intubation for anesthesia for abdominal surgery. In contrast with patient who have cancer, these patients have a good life expectancy. The treatment decision may have consequences for the quality of their lives for many years. Most of the procedures are elective: patients are rarely in a life-threatening condition. It is justified to consult colleagues from other departments and seek advice from experienced experts before placing a stent.

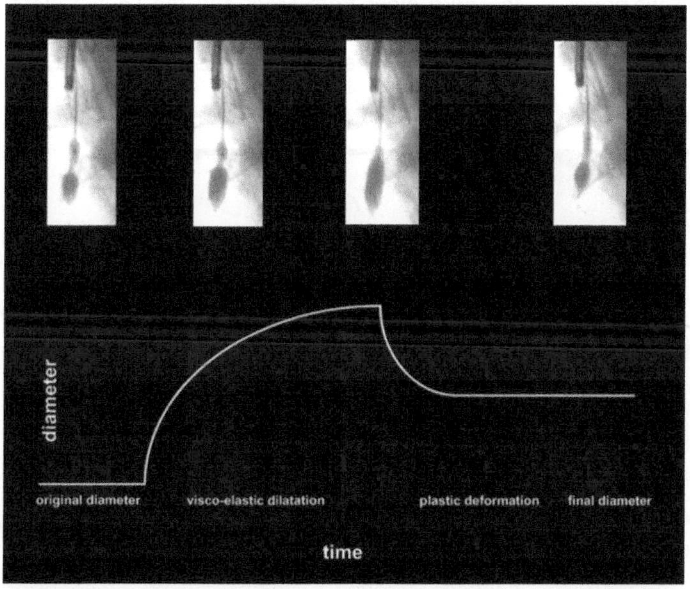

Fig. 11. Strictured tissue structures have viscoelastoplastic behavior. If dilatation pressure is applied (eg, with balloon dilatation), it takes a while until the stenosis opens (viscous). If the dilatation pressure is released, an elastic part recovers and shrinking occurs but the stenosis remains partially open (plastic deformation).

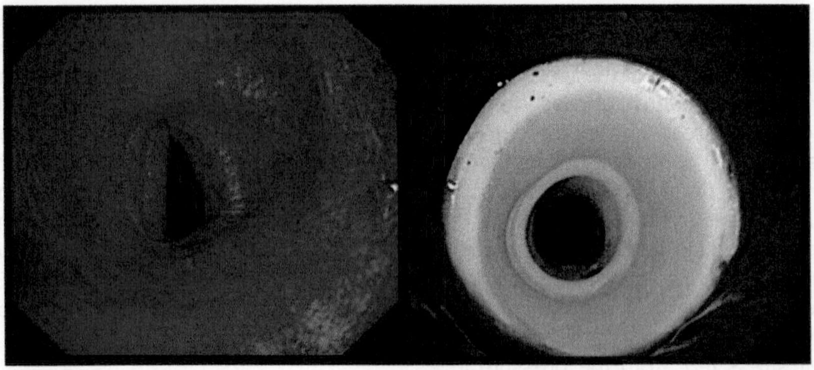

Fig. 12. An hourglass-shaped benign stricture (*left*) is treated with a Vergnon silicone stent (*right*).

As mentioned earlier, there are several types of stents. Silicone stents have the best safety record. Standard stents such as the Dumon stents are not always ideal for stenosis of the trachea. Benign stenoses are often triangular shaped in one plane and hourglass shaped in the other plane. With the exception of the anatomically shaped Dynamic stent, they are all round and cylindrical. The hoop stress (expansion force) that is necessary to counteract the constricting force is not equally distributed over the inner surface of the narrowed trachea, which results in higher pinpoint pressures at the most narrowed part. Unless a stent can adapt properly, the mucosa and the cartilages can be harmed further. In biomechanical terms, a stent is a long-term dilatator and the previously mentioned principles of viscoelastoplasticity apply. The stent is held in place by friction only. If the stricture opens gradually, wall contact pressure decreases and the stent can migrate. In benign stenoses, migration rates of up to 30% have been reported. For those stenoses, we prefer the Vergnon stent, which is a modified Dumon stent with larger diameters at the ends. It adapts better to the hourglass shape than the normal cylindrical stent (**Fig. 12**).

Less often, migration is encountered with self-expanding metal stents. These stents are even easier to place than silicone stents. They can be implanted with flexible bronchoscopes, either under direct vision or with fluoroscopic control. General anesthesia is not necessary and no special instruments are required. Most metal stents are made from nitinol, a shape-memory alloy that has some unique properties. Nitinol stents open a stricture slowly because of their structure and their specific memory ability. The metal stents that are currently used adapt well to benign strictures because the moving filaments can reshape better than silicone stents (**Fig. 13**).

The commonly used Ultraflex stent from Boston Scientific is partially covered. Soon after deployment, the uncovered ends are embedded in the mucosa, which prevents migration but makes removal difficult. Other metallic stents, such as the Aero stent from Merit and the Leufen stent, are fully covered. Removal is easier, but migration is common. The upper part of the trachea is a

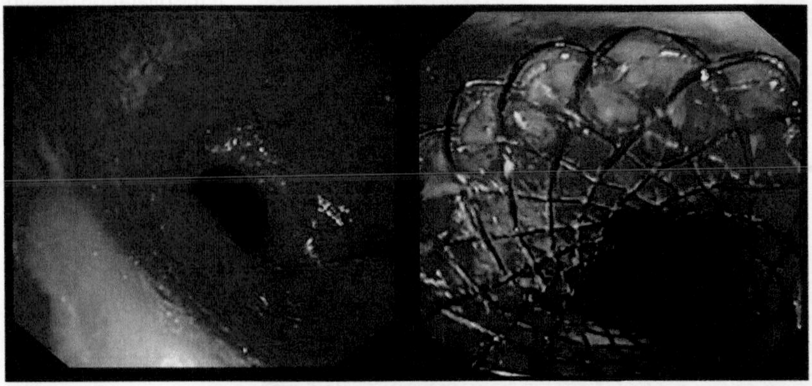

Fig. 13. If a silicone stent cannot be placed (*left*), a self-expanding metal stent (*right*) is an alternative, but more potential complications have to be expected.

delicate area. The high pressure necessary to prevent migration bears the risk of peribronchial inflammation with temporary or even permanent damage to the recurrent nerve. Losing speech ability is a serious impairment of a patient's quality of life. This complication of stent placement should be avoided with all possible means. One feasible option to prevent stent migration is fixation. We either fix these high tracheal stents with sutures through the skin or inside the trachea with a dedicated set of instruments, as shown in **Fig. 12**. A long needle holder and a knot pusher enables any stent to be sutured to the posterior membrane (**Fig. 14**).[25]

Besides migration, the other 2 common complications of stent treatment are mucus plugging and granulation tissue formation. Problems with retained secretions are often seen in smokers or patients with chronic infections and in patients who are too weak to cough efficiently. Despite all efforts of surface treatment, mucus sticks to the inner lumen of all commercially available stents. In addition to impairing airflow, these mucous layers and membranes are colonized with various kinds of bacteria and fungi. Biofilms are a source of recurrent infections and the smell has consequences for the social life of a patient to a similar degree as impaired speaking ability. Although halitosis is not life threatening, it can severely impair a patient's well-being. The most important countermeasure against mucus buildup and halitosis is mist inhalation. Every patient with an airway stent must get a prescription for an appropriate inhalation device.

The third complication of stent placement is the most troublesome. Stents are foreign bodies and they irritate the mucosa. They impair local blood flow, they scratch the surface, they are a reservoir for bacteria, and they cause galvanic currents where their metal touches the mucosa. All these factors contribute to the formation of granulation tissue. Fatigue fractures with broken wires that spike into the tissue are the strongest stimuli for this adverse reaction (**Fig. 15**).

Granulation tissue that develops at the ends of stents often narrows the lumen of the airway more than the original disorder. Stent-induced strictures are so common that the US Food and Drug Administration released a warning against the use of metal stents in benign diseases.[26] A typical scenario is that newly developed stenoses at the edges of a stent are treated with 1 or 2 other stents, making the problem worse. It is the responsibility of physicians to be cautious when making treatment decisions. Industry partners are challenged to develop better stents. At present, we advocate restricting the use of metallic stents to those few cases in which all other options have been exhausted.

If granulation tissue obstructs the lumen it can be removed with any endoscopic cutting technique, such as laser photocoagulation or APC. Some stents are inflammable and we recommend the use of cryotherapy because it eliminates the risk of ignition hazards. As a preventive measure, antiproliferating drugs or radiation therapy can be administered. These measures do not break up collagen but only act on doubling cells. There are

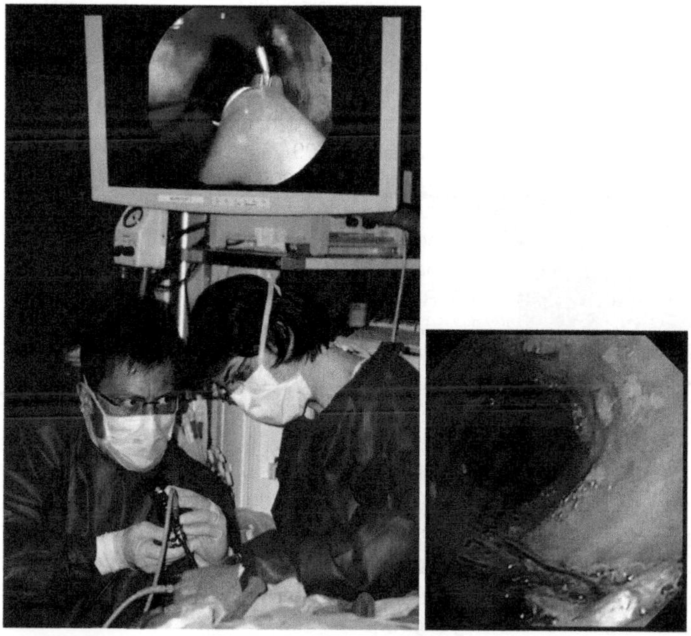

Fig. 14. Dr Stefan Welter sutures a stent endoscopically to the posterior membrane (*inset*) in order to prevent stent migration.

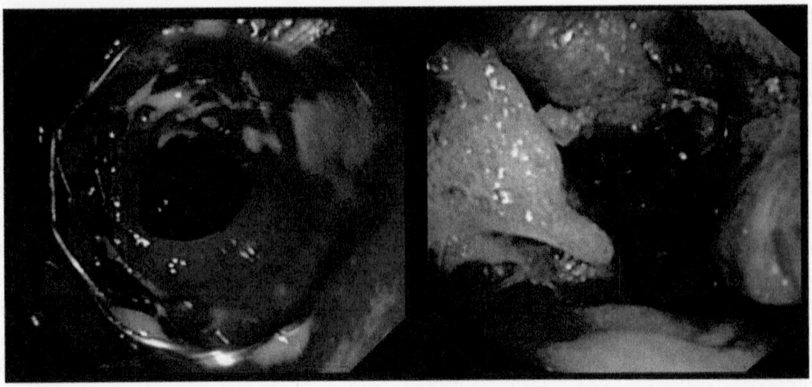

Fig. 15. Granulation tissue and scars often develop at the edges of metallic stents (*left*). Growth of granulation tissue and fractured wires of metal stents obstruct the tracheal lumen (*right*).

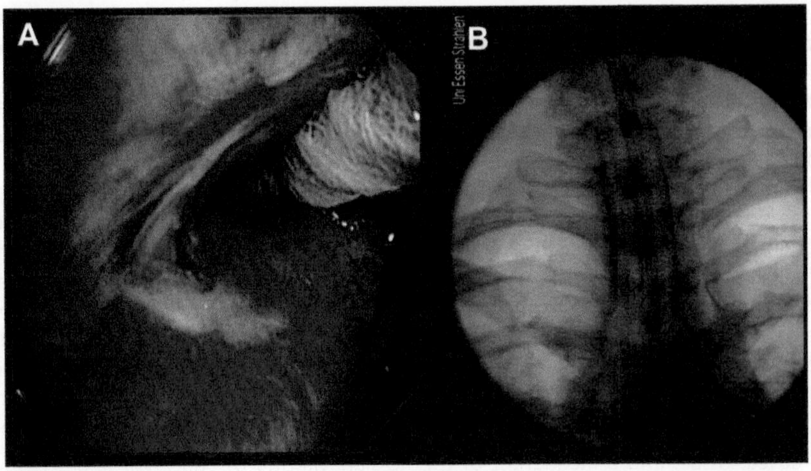

Fig. 16. Topical application of Mitomycin (*A*) or brachytherapy (*B*) are the most commonly used methods for preventing regrowth of granulation tissue.

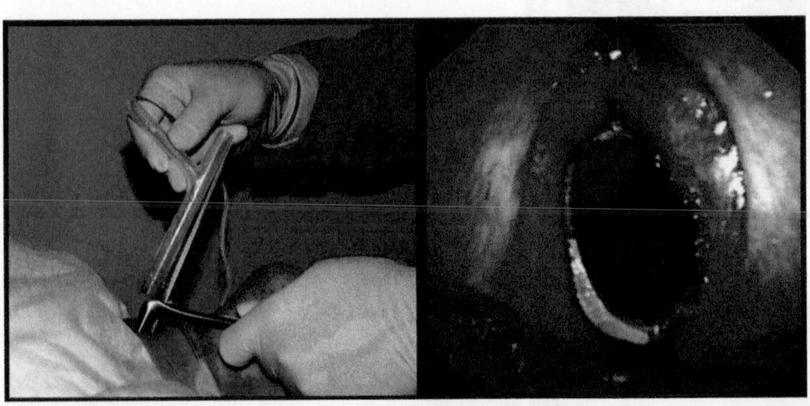

Fig. 17. For very high tracheal stenosis, a Montgomery T-tube, inserted under bronchoscopic control (*left*) is still the safest option. It enables breathing, speaking, and suctioning (*right*).

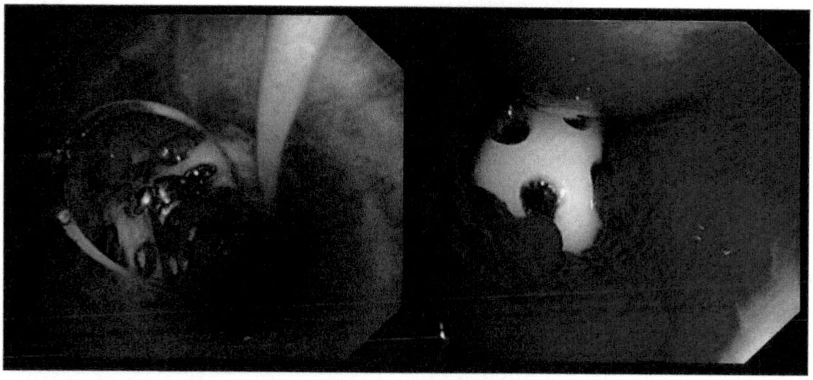

Fig. 18. If everything else fails and if chronic intractable inflammation narrows the tracheal lumen, a speech cannula is used to provide airway patency with acceptable quality of life.

no controlled studies so our recommendations are based on cases reports and clinical observations. Immediately after removal of granulation tissue, we apply mitomycin topically on the mucosa or give brachytherapy (7.5 Gy 1 or 2 times).[27–29] The use of locally administered corticosteroids might have beneficial effects as well.[30] It seems that these regimens work without noticeable side effects (**Fig. 16**).

It has already been mentioned that the upper third part of the trachea is a danger zone for the use of indwelling stents. For very high stenoses, extending up to the cricoid, we prefer Montgomery T-tubes. This technique requires a tracheotomy, which makes it less attractive than inner tracheal stents. However, T-tubes are safer, because patients can suck out their mucus at any time. These stents are not held in place by wall pressure, have fewer side effects, and can be exchanged easily (**Fig. 17**).[31]

In addition, there are patients with destroyed tracheas, active inflammation, and swelling that reaches up to the vocal chords. Under these circumstances, a well-fitting tracheal speech cannula is sometimes the best solution. If such a cannula is ordered properly and placed under bronchoscopic control, making sure that the speech holes are accurately positioned, it can be a reasonable alternative to surgery or stent placement. Whether plastic prostheses or a silver cannula are used does not matter. The main purpose is to provide enough airflow, retain speech, and let patients care for themselves without dependence on others (**Fig. 18**).

At the time of writing there are many scientific groups and industry partners working on better solutions. Drug-releasing stents, stents that apply low-dose radiation, biodegradable stents, and so forth will be available in the near future. A few months ago, a team of doctors manufactured a tailored plastic stent for a child with a malacic bronchus on a personal three-dimensional printer.[32] Individualized therapy is the most appropriate and should also be applied to patients with tracheal stenoses. Patients deserve an interdisciplinary approach to their problems.

REFERENCES

1. Freitag L, Ernst A, Unger M, et al. A proposed classification system of central airway stenosis. Eur Respir J 2007;30(1):7–12.
2. Theegarten D, Freitag L. Scar carcinoma of the trachea after tracheotomy. Case report and review of the literature. Respiration 1993;60(4):250–3.
3. Zimmermann C, Freitag L, Schönhofer B. Undetected tracheal tumours responsible for ventilator-dependency. Dtsch Med Wochenschr 2002; 127(10):497–9.
4. Bolliger CT, Sutedja TG, Strausz J, et al. Therapeutic bronchoscopy with immediate effect: laser, electrocautery, argon plasma coagulation and stents. Eur Respir J 2006;27(6):1258–71.
5. Micaud G. Malignant central airway obstruction. In: Ernst A, Herth F, editors. Principles and practice of interventional pulmonology. Springer Science; 2013. p. 259–68.
6. Dumon MC, Cavaliere S, Dumon JF. Endobronchial laser therapy. Rev Mal Respir 1999;16:601–8.
7. Boxem T, Muller M, Venmanns B, et al. ND-YAG laser vs bronchoscopic electrocautery for palliation of symptomatic airway obstruction: a cost-effectiveness study. Chest 1999;116:1108–12.
8. Freitag L, Reichle G. Argon plasma coagulation. In: Beamis J, Mathur P, Mehta AC, editors. Interventional pulmonary medicine. Marcel Decker; 2004. p. 203–13.
9. Reddy C, Majid A, Michaud G, et al. Gas embolism following bronchoscopic argon plasma coagulation. Chest 2008;134(5):1066–9.
10. Homasson JP, Renault P, Angebault M, et al. Bronchoscopic cryotherapy for airway strictures caused by tumors. Chest 1986;90:159–64.

11. Vergnon JM, Boucheron S, Bonamour D, et al. Intratracheal destruction of tumor lesions: laser or cryotherapy? Rev Pneumol Clin 1987;43:19–25.
12. Freitag L, Ernst A, Thomas M, et al. Sequential photodynamic therapy (PDT) and high dose brachytherapy for endobronchial tumour control in patients with limited bronchogenic carcinoma. Thorax 2004; 59(9):790–3.
13. Celikoglu F, Celikoglu SI, Goldberg EP. Bronchoscopic intratumoral chemotherapy of lung cancer. Lung Cancer 2008;61(1):1–12.
14. Hohenforst-Schmidt W, Zarogoulidis P, Darwiche K, et al. Intratumoral chemotherapy for lung cancer: re-challenge current targeted therapies. Drug Des Devel Ther 2013;7:571–83.
15. Anantham D. Management principles of nonmalignant airway obstructions. In: Ernst A, Herth F, editors. Principles and practice of interventional pulmonology. Springer Science; 2013. p. 269–83.
16. Freitag L. Airway stents. In: Strausz J, Bolliger CT, editors. Interventional pulmonology, European respiratory monograph. 2010;48:190–217.
17. Freitag L, Tekolf E, Stamatis G, et al. Clinical evaluation of a new bifurcated dynamic airway stent: a 5-year experience with 135 patients. Thorac Cardiovasc Surg 1997;45(1):6–12.
18. Karagiannidis C, Velehorschi V, Obertrifter B, et al. High-level expression of matrix-associated transforming growth factor-beta1 in benign airway stenosis. Chest 2006;129(5):1298–304.
19. Freitag L, Firusian N, Stamatis G, et al. The role of bronchoscopy in pulmonary complications due to mustard gas inhalation. Chest 1991; 100(5):1436–41.
20. Colt H, Murgu S. Post intubation tracheal stenosis. In: Bronchoscopy and central airway disorders. Elsevier Saunders; 2012. p. 95–103.
21. Amat B, Esselmann A, Reichle G, et al. The electrosurgical knife in an optimized intermittent cutting mode for the endoscopic treatment of benign web-like tracheobronchial stenosis. Arch Bronconeumol 2012;48(1):14–21.
22. Venhaus M, Behn C, Freitag L, et al. Simulations and experiments of the balloon dilatation of airway stenoses. Biomed Tech 2009;54(4):187–95.
23. Shitrit D, Kuchuk M, Zismanov V, et al. Bronchoscopic balloon dilatation of tracheobronchial stenosis: long-term follow-up. Eur J Cardiothorac Surg 2010;38(2):198–202.
24. Noppen M. Bronchoscopic balloon dilatation in the combined management of postintubation stenosis of the trachea in adults. Chest 1997;112:1136–40.
25. Welter S, Jacobs J, Krbek T, et al. A new endoscopic technique for intraluminal repair of posterior tracheal laceration. Ann Thorac Surg 2010;90(2):686–8.
26. Food and Drug Administration public health notification: complications from metallic stents in patients with benign airway disorders. 2009. Available at: www.fda.gov/MedicalDevicesSafety/AlertsandNotices/.
27. Rhabarb R, Shapsay SM, Healy GB. Mitomycin effects on laryngeal and tracheal stenosis, benefits and complications. Ann Otol Rhinol Laryngol 2001; 110:1–6.
28. Kennedy A, Sonett J, Orens J. High dose rate brachytherapy to prevent recurrent benign hyperplasia in lung transplant bronchi: theoretical and clinical considerations. J Heart Lung Transplant 2000;19:155–9.
29. Kramer MR, Katz A, Yarmolovsky A. Successful use of high dose rate brachytherapy for non-malignant bronchial obstruction. Thorax 2001;56:415–6.
30. Hoffmann GS, Thomas-Golbanov CK, Chan J, et al. Treatment of subglottic stenosis, due to Wegener's granulomatosis, with intralesional corticosteroids and dilatation. J Rheumatol 2003;30(5):1017–21.
31. Montgomery W. T-tube tracheal stent. Arch Otolaryngol 1965;82:320–1.
32. Zopf DA, Nelson ME, Ohye R, et al. Bioresorbable airway splint created with a three-dimensional printer. N Engl J Med 2013;368:2043–5.

Repair of Tracheobronchial Injuries

Stefan Welter

KEYWORDS

• Tracheobronchial injury • Airway management • Iatrogenic tracheal laceration
• Mediastinal emphysema

KEY POINTS

- Establishment of a secure airway is the first step in the management of non-iatrogenic tracheobronchial injuries followed by control and repair of vascular and other life threatening associated injuries.
- Operative tracheobronchial reconstruction is mandatory in penetrating injuries and when there is associated esophageal injury or mediastinitis is evident.
- Conservative treatment in patients with incomplete tracheal membrane laceration (TML) and case-by-case decision making in full-thickness TML is recommended, depending on the severity of the accompanying problems and patient condition.
- Endotracheal reconstruction of TML could be a possibility in experienced centers in the future for all patients who tolerate jet ventilation.

Videos of complete intraluminal repair of a iatrogenic tracheal laceration and expiratory tracheal collapse in the region of a former tracheal membrane laceration accompany this article at http://www.thoracic.theclinics.com/

INTRODUCTION

Tracheobronchial injuries (TBIs) are a heterogeneous group of injuries in terms of the trauma mechanism, anatomic site of damage, and severity of subsequent respiratory complications (**Table 1**).[1] TBIs are often life threatening and require early and skillful airway management, careful evaluation, and qualified operative repair, which is best offered in thoracic surgery units.[2] The most important discrimination of TBI is traumatic damage versus iatrogenic tracheal laceration. Iatrogenic tracheal lacerations are rarely accompanied by esophagus rupture, whereas blunt or penetrating injuries of the tracheobronchial tree are most often accompanied by a variety of different and sometimes life-threatening injuries.[3] Therefore, the 2 types of injury are described separately in this article. Intubation-associated injuries and blunt trauma account for the most events in the Western countries. Penetrating injuries predominate in war zones.

NONIATROGENIC TBI

Statistics

Blunt and penetrating injuries often occur with other injuries, especially those of the great vessels; without early recognition and prompt intervention, they are frequently fatal. The prognoses of patients who reach hospital mainly depend on airway management and the extent of associated injuries. Blunt trauma is most frequently (59%) caused by motor vehicle accidents, and the mortality is around 9%.[4] The incidence of TBI after blunt trauma is low (2.8%), as was found in a postmortem analysis by Bertelsen and Howitz.[5] Another study showed an even lower incidence of 0.5%.[6] Of all the blunt TBI cases reviewed by Symbas

This work was not funded. There is no conflict of interest to disclose.
Department of Thoracic Surgery and Endoscopy, Ruhrlandklinik, University Clinic, University of Duisburg-Essen, Tüschener Weg 40, Essen 45239, Germany
E-mail address: stefan.welter@ruhrlandklinik.uk-essen.de

Thorac Surg Clin 24 (2014) 41–50
http://dx.doi.org/10.1016/j.thorsurg.2013.10.006

Table 1
Pathomechanism of tracheobronchial injuries

Blunt trauma	Traffic accident	Dashboard injury, deceleration with shoulder belt
	Burying	Thoracic compression
	Fall	Deceleration, direct cervical injury
	Crush injury	Compression, rib fractures, cartilage fractures
	Hyperextension of the cervical trachea	Distraction injury, laryngotracheal separation
Penetrating injury	Gunshot	Transmission of kinetic energy
	Stabbing	Sharp tissue transection
Iatrogenic	Intraoperative	Excision of wall structures, devascularization
	Postintubation	Direct longitudinal laceration

and colleagues,[7] 136 (71%) had transverse ruptures, 33 (18%) had longitudinal ruptures, and 14 (8%) had complex ruptures. Almost 75% to 80% of penetrating injuries involve the cervical trachea, whereas 75% to 80% of blunt injuries occur within 2.5 cm of the carina and 43% occur within the first 2 cm of the right main bronchus.[4,7] Intrathoracic blunt TBI is regularly associated with other organ involvement.[8] Thus, 80% of accident victims with evidence of TBI die before reaching hospital.[9] The distribution of TBIs in Germany was described by Schneider and colleagues[2]; 58% were iatrogenic and 41% were traumatic in origin. From the 429 cases of noniatrogenic origin, 276 (64%) were caused by blunt trauma, 94 (22%) had penetrating injuries, and 16 (4%) had gunshot injuries in a 5-year observation period. All bullet injuries and 82% of penetrating injuries were treated operatively. Penetrating thoracic injuries are also often associated with other injuries. Inci and colleagues[10] found, in a series of 755 trauma patients, 190 cases with hemothorax, 184 cases with hemopneumothorax, 144 cases with pneumothorax, and nearly 150 patients with rupture of the diaphragm or other injuries.

Mechanisms of Noniatrogenic Tracheobronchial Injury and Pathology

The bronchial tree and the lower two-thirds of the trachea have good bony protection, whereas the cervical trachea is exposed anteriorly. Therefore, lesions of the cervical trachea occur after sharp or blunt trauma to the anterior or lateral aspect or hyperextension of the neck.[5] Injuries of the thoracic trachea or main bronchi resulting from blunt trauma might be explained by 3 models[11]:

- A sudden increase in the airway pressure when the glottis is closed may lead to tracheal perforation or rupture of the main bronchi. This mechanism may explain TBI after blunt abdominal injury with sudden displacement of the diaphragm.
- Extensive anteroposterior chest compression forcing the lungs apart laterally and causing distention and rupture of central airway structures near the carina.
- Rapid deceleration with shearing force applied to the fixed portions of the trachea at the junctions to the cricoid or the carina may cause rupture of the mobile portions of the trachea.

Blunt TBIs are associated with major accompanying injuries in 40% to 100% of cases, primarily involving orthopedic, facial, pulmonary, and intra-abdominal injuries, which may be the primary determinant in patient outcome.[8,12] Stab wounds or gunshot wounds of the lower trachea or carina are almost absent in hospitals because they may be associated with fatal injuries of the heart or great vessels and would never arrive in trauma centers for resuscitation.[12] Major accompanying injuries, mainly of the esophagus and great vessels, were reported for in 50% to 80% of penetrating TBIs.[12]

Diagnostics

The diagnosis of TBI can be missed initially, especially in patients with other organ injuries.[13,14] Clinical signs of TBI are listed in **Box 1**. Tachypnea and subcutaneous emphysema are the most common. If TBI is suspected, chest roentgenogram is the first step in diagnosis. Pneumothorax and pneumomediastinum are common in patients with intrathoracic rather than cervical tracheal injuries.[15] Other possible injuries associated with TBIs are listed in **Box 2**. Occasionally, complete or near-complete transection of major bronchi results in the "fallen lung" sign on chest radiographs, which refers to the collapsed lung in a dependent position, hanging on the hilum only by its vascular attachments. Placement of a tube thoracostomy

Box 1
Clinical signs of noniatrogenic tracheobronchial injury

- Air escaping from a neck wound
- Massive air leak after placement of a tube thoracostomy
- Persistent lung collapse despite adequate drainage
- Hemoptysis
- Stridor
- Cyanosis
- Subcutaneous emphysema
- Progressive dyspnea and tachypnea, respiratory distress
- Dysphagia

Data from Refs.[12,14,16]

can be the immediate consequence. A chest computed tomography (CT) is mainly helpful for evaluating associated injuries, which are present in almost 75% of patients with blunt TBI.[12,16] On the other hand, a CT scan is used in patients with severe multisystem trauma and has been proved to be useful in detecting unexpected thoracic injuries.[17] With a high index of suspicion, TBI can be identified on CT scans by paratracheal air (93%), deep cervical emphysema, and pneumomediastinum (100%) in every patient with TBI.[15] Direct visualization of the tracheal wall injury is less reliable (71%). Defects or discontinuity, local wall deformity, or tracheal ring fractures (14%) can be identified in some cases.[15] Altogether, suspicious tracheal injury can be identified in 85% to 100% of chest CT scans.[18] On the other hand, all these signs may have other causes so they are not evidentiary for TBI.

Bronchoscopy is the most important procedure to exactly locate and assess TBI. It can be used for guidance of the intubation tube in critically ill patients.[19,20] The diagnosis of TBI can also be established with rigid bronchoscopy[14] because it allows bronchial clearance, removal of blood clots, and exact measurement of the lesion.

Box 2
Injuries often associated with traumatic tracheobronchial injuries

- Pneumothorax
- Hemothorax
- Rib fractures
- Pulmonary contusion and parenchymal rupture
- Laryngeal fractures and recurrent laryngeal nerve injury
- Esophageal injury
- Injury of the cervical spine and spinal cord
- Injury of intrathoracic great vessels and pulmonary artery and heart injuries
- Vascular injury of the carotid arteries and jugular veins

Data from Inci I, Ozçelik C, Taçyildiz I, et al. Penetrating chest injuries: unusually high incidence of high-velocity gunshot wounds in civilian practice. World J Surg 1998;22:438–42; and Mussi A, Ambrogi MC, Ribechini A, et al. Acute major airway injuries: clinical features and management. Eur J Cardiothorac Surg 2001;20:46–52.

Management

Early airway assessment followed by definitive airway protection is the key to neck trauma management[21] and TBI. The standard technique is direct laryngoscopy followed by rapid sequence intubation of the patient with shock, hypoxia, predicted operative need, or obvious airway compromise. Progressive edema and swelling of the larynx, as well as progressive mediastinal emphysema or bleeding, can make intubation unfeasible. In this situation, a delay in airway protection with a tracheal tube is dangerous. Emergency tracheal intubation is preferably performed with the use of succinylcholine.[22] On the other hand, it is better to bring a patient with spontaneous respiration alive into hospital, than converting a partial airway obstruction into a complete obstruction by an unskilled attempt to place a tracheal tube.[14]

To establish a secure airway, exposed parts of the trachea, eg, with a stab wound of the upper third of the trachea, are best intubated through the wound. After local debridement, this can be used as midterm treatment as well.[14,16,20,21]

Cricotomy or tracheostomy is the required procedure when laryngeal anatomy is altered or other attempts have failed to secure the airway.[20] This situation occurs especially when there is associated extensive maxillofacial damage. In such case, tracheostomy is the only way to identify tracheal injury and secure the airway.

Operative Repair

Patients with small injuries, poor clinical and radiological manifestation, or no appreciable leaks, who do not require positive pressure ventilation and are nonprogressive, may be treated nonoperatively.[20,23,24] These cases need to be thoroughly monitored so that any appearing stridor, dyspnea, or other consequences of TBI can be treated immediately.

For all other cases, primary surgical repair represents the treatment of choice, especially in noniatrogenic TBI, to reestablish airway continuity.[19,20] Most TBIs can be repaired using established principles of airway surgery and anesthesia.[7] Sparing debridement and primary repair with 3-0 or 4-0 absorbable sutures are used for blunt as well as penetrating TBI.[16,20,24] Transverse ruptures are best adapted with interrupted sutures where the knots lie outside the wall, and longitudinal ruptures may be repaired with continuous suture.[7] Covering with tissue flaps is usually not necessary, but if the blood supply is impaired after a massive trauma, pericardial or mediastinal fat flaps might be helpful to prevent dehiscence. As described by Grillo and colleagues,[25] tracheal dissection around the lesion must be performed meticulously and closed along the trachea to minimize the risk for laryngeal nerve injury. If significant tracheobronchial damage is obvious, circumferential resection with end-to-end anastomosis while preserving the blood supply is preferable to partial debridement with attempted primary repair.[12,25,26] In this situation, high-frequency ventilation with the tip of the orotracheal tube positioned cephalad to the rupture and only the gas inflow catheter passing into the distal airway is helpful and provides an unobstructed operative field and good gas exchange.[7,12] This technique is well established in elective tracheal surgery. Only extensive injuries of the carina should be repaired rather than resected, if possible.[12] Unfortunately, late sequela with fibrous obstruction is possible.[7]

The diagnosis of TBI after blunt trauma is sometimes delayed, with a median time of 6 months.[13] Granulation tissue formation or later formation of fibrotic stricture leads to obstructive complications. Dyspnea and pneumonia are the most common complaints in such cases. Bronchial sleeve resections of stenotic parts with end-to-end anastomosis can be performed safely in most situations using standard techniques of lung cancer resection (**Fig. 1**).[13,25,26]

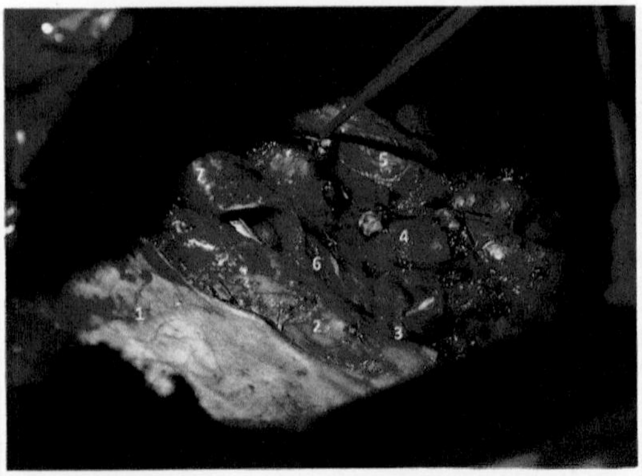

Fig. 1. Accessible structures through a right posterolateral thoracotomy. View through a right posterolateral thoracotomy that was performed for a central right main bronchus stenosis. Sleeve resection of the upper lobe with parts of the posterolateral tracheal wall and end-to-end anastomosis of the intermediate bronchus with the trachea was performed to completely remove the obstructing tissue. The white numbers are: 1, spine; 2, esophagus; 3, intermediate bronchus; 4, main right pulmonary artery; 5, superior vena cava; 6, left main bronchus; 7, distal trachea.

Penetrating Injuries

Immediate exploration of penetrating neck wounds is crucial for survival because vascular and esophageal injuries are frequent and the tracheal injury often includes cartilages as well as ligamentous portions.[8,15] With the establishment of a secure airway, the next step is control or repair of vascular damages. With the help of an experienced vascular surgeon, adequate cerebral perfusion might be restored, but is not always indicated, when ischemia has already caused major brain damage.[21] The next step is an evaluation of the esophagus and the trachea. Combined injuries of the trachea and the hypopharynx or esophagus also need early and primary repair.[27] After a meticulous debridement, the reparation of the esophagus is performed in 2 layers and the trachea is separately reconstructed. Even horizontal transection of the esophagus can be repaired with double-layer suture.[20] Both suture lines must be secured with the interposition of viable muscle, eg, strap muscle, mediastinal fatty tissue, or thymus gland,[14] to prevent later trachea-esophageal fistula. Primary wound closure at the end, under antibiotic protection is currently well established.

Surgical exploration and debridement followed by reconstruction of laryngotracheal injuries and primary wound closure has even been reported for war injuries with inflicted bomb fragments.[3,27,28] Whenever the glottis function is unclear, a protective, small-sized tracheostomy tube can be inserted 2 rings below the suture line.[14] Shotgun injuries need special attention, because the projectile produces a permanent cavity as a result of the crushing of the tissue as the projectile passes through, and a temporary cavity due to the expansion of the tissue particles away from the pathway of the bullet. This temporary cavity is much larger and needs to be assessed to understand the full extent of the injury. Hence, there is always a certain amount of disrupted and thermal damaged tissue around the visible bullet canal. High-velocity projectiles leave a much larger wound cavity than low-velocity projectiles from handguns.[12]

Operative Access

Injuries of the cervical trachea can be approached through a collar incision.[12] A good view and transcervical repair is possible for the upper two-thirds from a cervical approach with t-shape incision.[29] Moreover, splitting the manubrium down to the second intercostal space provides better exposure to the innominate artery and vein. When the exposure of a hemithorax or the mediastinum is necessary, median sternotomy is reasonable.[16] A bilateral thoracosternotomy (Clamshell incision) provides a good exposure to the mediastinum and both hemithoraces but provides no advantage for airway repair. Therefore, its use depends on the importance of the associated injuries.[12] Avulsions and ruptures of the right main bronchus, the carina, and the central part of the left main bronchus can be reached over a right anterolateral or posterolateral thoracotomy (**Fig. 2**).[16,26]

Discussion

With the need for early and precise airway management, beginning at the place of the accident, traumatic TBI differs greatly from iatrogenic TBI. Both penetrating and blunt TBI are frequently associated with the involvement of other organs, and some of them are fatal before a trauma center is reached.[5,10,12] The prognosis of iatrogenic TBI with adequate management depends mainly on the comorbidities, rather than the injuries. Acute clinical awareness is essential for rapid diagnosis and successful surgical intervention in all patients with TBI.[3,16] Airway protection for patients with respiratory instability is best achieved with orotracheal intubation and, if possible, it should always be performed guided by bronchoscopy, in order to avoid extension of the injury.[20] The liberal use of early flexible bronchoscopy must be encouraged; it is the only way to confirm the diagnosis and allows determination of the location, extent, and depth of the lesion.[16,20] Many iatrogenic tracheal lacerations can be treated conservatively, whereas almost all traumatic TBIs need early operative reconstruction, which must be adjusted to the associated injuries.[3] Operative access and the techniques for reconstruction are familiar to the thoracic surgeon because they are similar to the techniques used in airway resection and reconstruction for benign and malign diseases.[26] Thoracic surgery experts play the key role in the management of the injured airway.[14] Therefore, Farzanegan and colleagues[14]

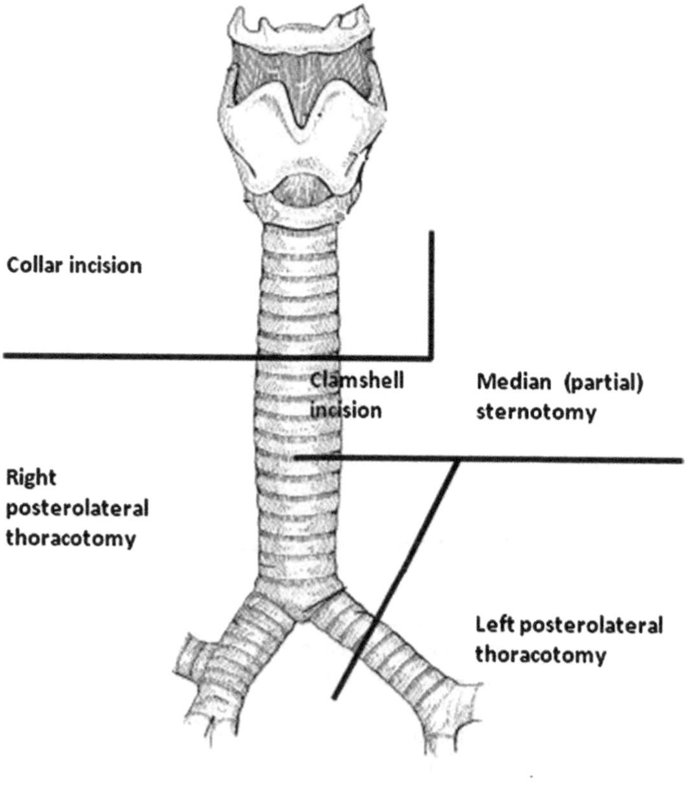

Fig. 2. Scheme of access to the tracheobronchial tree. Operative access to different regions of the trachea and main bronchi. With the right posterolateral thoracotomy, the whole right bronchial system, the carina, and the distal trachea as well as the left central main bronchus are accessible.

recommend protection of the airway as the first measure and referring the patient for definitive treatment to a specialist department.

IATROGENIC TML

Introduction

Iatrogenic TML is a rare direct complication of endotracheal intubation, percutaneous dilatational tracheostomy, and rigid bronchoscopy, with an incidence of 0.05% to 0.5%.[2] Some high-risk situations are well known, such as emergency intubation, intubation by unskilled persons, use and late removal of a stylet during intubation, manipulation of the tube with blocked cuff, and the use of high-pressure cuffs.[15,30] Dilatational tracheostomy is a risk when the procedure is not controlled with bronchoscopy, the introduction is not in the midline, or the bougie is pushed through a cartilage ring rather than the membrane in between.[31] Also, there are patient-specific risk factors, such as female gender, age between 50 and 70 years, a high body mass index, and long-term use of corticoids. It most often includes the posterior wall in the midline or right paramedian and can reach into the right main bronchus.[2,32,33]

Classification

Because treatment algorithms depend mainly on clinical problems after TML, there are 2 main categories that need to be evaluated and described:

1. The depth and length of the rupture and the severity, including accompanying injury of the esophagus; and
2. The severity of distant consequences, such as mediastinal emphysema, air leakage, and others.

A new morphologic classification, based on the lacerated layers of the tracheal membrane, was recently published by Cardillo.[34] Level I and level II TMLs are defined as superficial injuries in which the posterior plane of the trachea is not completely disrupted; level IIIa TMLs are defined as complete laceration of the tracheal wall with esophageal or mediastinal soft tissue hernia, without esophageal injury or mediastinitis; and level IIIb TMLs are defined as complete laceration with esophageal injury or mediastinitis.

Symptoms

The clinical symptoms are caused by local bleeding, by the mediastinal tissue protruding into the tracheal lumen, and by air leakage into the mediastinum of the right (rarely left) hemithorax (**Box 3**).

Box 3
Symptoms following TML

- Hemoptysis or blood in the tube after intubation is highly suspicious
- Expanding mediastinal and subcutaneous emphysema
- Pneumothorax and even tension pneumothorax are typical complications of TML
- Spontaneously breathing patients may have expiratory tracheal collapse leading to respiratory exhaustion with the need for reintubation
- A sudden rise in ventilatory pressure and bloating of the mediastinum when the tip of the ventilation tube slips into the lesion. This is a life-threatening emergency
- Massive air leak from the mouth in mechanically ventilated patients

Data from Marchese R, Mercadante S, Paglino G, et al. Tracheal stent to repair tracheal laceration after double-lumen intubation. Ann Thorac Surg 2012;94:1001–3; and Venkataramanappa V, Boujoukos AJ, Sakai T. The diagnostic challenge of a tracheal tear with a double-lumen endobronchial tube: massive air leak developing from the mouth during mechanical ventilation. J Clin Anesth 2011;23:66–70.

Diagnostics

Because a delay in proper treatment of the lesion, especially if there is accompanying esophageal injury, increases the risk for major complications and death,[14,27] a targeted program of procedures is necessary to verify the diagnosis, classify the lesion, and plan the treatment. Radiographic examination and CT of the chest reveal mediastinal and subcutaneous emphysema, pneumothorax, and enlarged tracheal diameter around the tube cuff.[15,18] The immediate measure might be the insertion of a thoracic drain. The next step is the bronchoscopic evaluation of the trachea, with simultaneous suction to clear the bronchial system of blood and secretions. A tube must be drawn back until the whole lesion is exposed. Superficial lesions might now be covered with fibrin to stop further bleeding.[34] If necessary, a tube can be pushed forward until the tip is safely distal from the lesion and the cuff is blocked as little as possible.

Treatment

Conservative treatment

Conservative treatment includes medication against tussive irritation, mild inspiratory pressures, noninvasive ventilatory support if necessary, intense physiotherapy to clear secretions, and possibly application of fibrin to cover the lesion.[34,35,36] This treatment allows both edges of the tracheal membrane to agglutinate with the mediastinal tissues behind and allows the development of a closed fibrin layer. Unfortunately, there are major doubts as to whether the laceration itself will heal together or the mediastinal contents will be covered with an epithelial layer over time and the muscular tracheal wall will remain retracted to both sides.

Operative treatment

Operative treatment includes complete anatomic restoration of the lesion with interrupted or running resorbable sutures.[32] Coverage of the lesion with an intercostal muscle flap[37] is possible, but seems to be unnecessary because the lesion most often heals without problems. However, it might support healing when mediastinitis is already evident. The surgical access depends on the region of the injury. For the upper half of the trachea, surgical repair via tracheostomy[38] or transcervical access with a tracheotomy[29,39] is described, whereas the lower half can be reached by a right posterolateral thoracotomy.[26,40,41] All these methods are described as effective, but they all need an additional surgical access. A new and promising, exclusively endoluminal repair of TML was recently published by Welter and colleagues.[33] With a newly developed optical needle holder (KARL STORZ GmBH & Co KG, Tuttlingen, Germany), a TML can be repaired with a running 2-0 Vicryl thread (UCLX-needle, Ethicon, Germany) under visual control (Video 1). This technique completely omits surgical incision and their possible long-term consequences. At present, this method can be applied to patients who tolerate jet ventilation and who have at least a small strip of membranous posterior wall on both sides to insert the needle into. At present, the authors have experience with 10 TMLs repaired with endotracheal suture. The operation duration was reduced from 115 minutes to 45 minutes or less, and no operative complications or mediastinitis has been found. All patients with TML, independent of the mode of treatment, should receive broad-spectrum antibiotics for a minimum of 5 days.

Treatment Decision

The decision for conservative or operative treatment is easy in some cases and difficult in others. Superficial TML without concomitant symptoms, analogous to level I and II lacerations according to the Cardillo classification,[34] are best treated conservatively, and additional injury of the esophagus (level IIIb lacerations) as well as the failure of conservative treatment need categorical operative intervention.[30,33] Full-thickness TML without esophageal injury (level IIIa laceration) can be managed with conservative or operative treatment, and in this situation, all concomitant local problems have to be taken into account: broad communication of the lesion with the pleural space, massive air leakage,[24] and pronounced mediastinal herniation in overweight patients (**Fig. 3**) are the major arguments for operative treatment. Smaller lesions, instability of the patient, a requirement for long-term ventilation independent of TML, no difficulties in completely bridging the lesion, and slim patients qualify for conservative treatment. In addition, medical risks for operative intervention have to be weighed against the advantage of anatomic reconstruction of the trachea in every individual situation. Endotracheal repair can be offered without increased morbidity to all patients who tolerate jet ventilation for a longer time and might be a better alternative to conservative treatment with prolonged ventilation.[33] In any case, full-thickness TML should be treated in specialized thoracic surgery units.

Discussion

Historically, TMLs have been classified by their location, length, and laterality. Cardillo and colleagues[34] first described a classification based on the anatomic layers that are disrupted by the

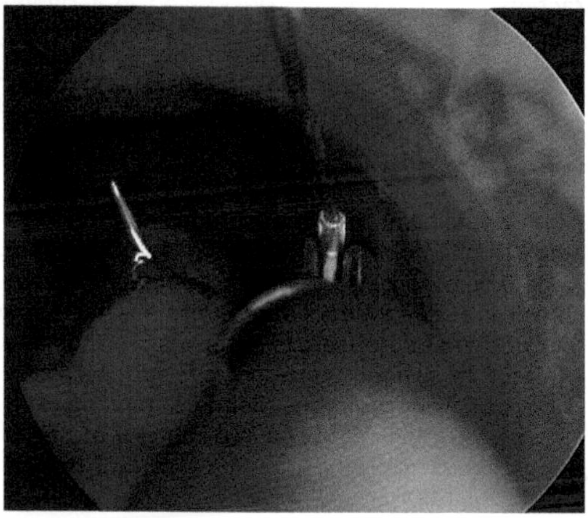

Fig. 3. Endoluminal protrusion of mediastinal fat through a tracheal membrane laceration. View in an overweight female patient with a tracheal membrane laceration after elective intubation for a knee arthroscopy. About 1 hour after extubation, reinsertion of the tracheal tube was necessary because of continuous cough, CO_2 retention, and prostration. Endotracheal suture was difficult but performed successfully in the end.

injury. Unfortunately, this anatomic classification is inconsequent, includes mediastinitis in the definition of a level IIIb laceration, and is not very helpful in clinical decision making. It is very simple to explain that incomplete TML does not need surgical intervention. Full-thickness rupture of the posterior tracheal wall is the lesion that needs experience-based decision making for conservative or operative treatment (**Table 2**). This decision can only be made with knowledge of the advantages and disadvantages of conservative and operative treatments: conservative treatment might be associated with lower mortality[32]; there is no additional scarring at the neck or thoracic wall, and there are no postthoracotomy complications.[33]

Cardillo and colleagues[34] recommend conservative treatment of level I–II TML and the management of level IIIa lesions in experienced institutions, based on their experience with 30 patients. The investigators covered all lesions with fibrin glue. Only 3 patients had level IIIa or IIIb lesions, which were the ones with collateral problems. One of them was successfully operated. At least these investigators have had only little experience for conservative treatment of full-thickness TML. Conti and colleagues[30] reported their experience with 28 patients with TML, including 8 with full-thickness TML, and all had initial conservative treatment. Several problems were described: 3 patients needed short-term noninvasive ventilation due to "mild respiratory distress," 2 needed operative relief of sterile mediastinal collections, and a tracheoesophageal fistula developed in 1 patient who needed lower esophageal exclusion. In 2 patients, bridging of the lesion was impossible; therefore, unilateral ventilation was necessary but was successful only in 1 patient. In 3 patients, "complete healing" took more than 1 month. In the end, 1 patient died as a consequence of TML and nonsurgical treatment. Another midterm consequence of nonoperative treatment recognized in our clinic is expiratory tracheal collapse because of respiratory insufficiency caused by mediastinal herniation (Video 2). This problem might be due to the detrimental effect of the clotting of both rims of the tracheal membrane with the mediastinal tissue from behind instead of healing together, which is especially problematic in patients with chronic obstructive pulmonary disease and in obese patients.

On the other hand, surgical repair is associated with increased mortality in some series.[32,41] This statement must be taken with care because often surgical repair is performed when conservative treatment has failed and thus there is no other alternative. Furthermore, surgery was performed in full-thickness lesions only and when the laceration was large. The author's group hold the impression that it does not make sense to compare these surgical results against series with conservative treatment including superficial lesions, small lesions, and easy-to-bridge lesions. Mortality is usually the consequence of underlying diseases.[30,33,41] Surgical repair allows an immediate anatomic restoration and closure of tracheopleural fistulation and prevents mediastinitis. This goal is reached in 100% of patients in some series.[42] However, surgical treatment requires a neck incision or a thoracotomy. With every collar incision, the trachea also has to be opened to gain access to the lesion.[29,38] Later, development of strictures is possible. Thoracotomy may require extensive adhesiolysis and is a risk for postoperative bleeding, infection, and postthoracotomy pain syndrome. This dilemma might be solved in the

Table 2
Treatment decision (TML): conservative versus operative and endotracheal

Clinical Situation	Conservative	Operative	Endotracheal
Esophageal involvement		X	
Broad communication with pleural space		X	X
Massive air leakage		X	X
Pronounced mediastinal herniation		X	X
Extension into right main bronchus		X	X
Increased medical risk	X		X
Jet ventilation not tolerated	X	X	
Small lesions	X		X
Superficial tracheal membrane laceration	X		X
Long-term ventilation required	X		X

future with more frequent use of endotracheal suture that allows anatomic restoration of the tracheal wall by omitting any surgical incision.[33]

Silicon stents are sporadically described to be effective in treating life-threatening TML.[43,44] However, because stents were developed to hold open the lumen of hollow organs, although they might seal a long laceration in some situations, they might also prevent the trachea from healing in a normal diameter. Furthermore, sputum expectoration is hampered, which often necessitates invasive procedures to remove the secretions.[42]

SUMMARY

The authors recommend conservative treatment in patients with incomplete TML and case-by-case decision making in full-thickness TML, depending on the severity of accompanying problems and patient condition. Endotracheal reconstruction could be a possibility in experienced centers in the future for all patients who tolerate jet ventilation. Operative reconstruction is mandatory when there is associated esophageal injury or mediastinitis is evident.

SUPPLEMENTARY DATA

Supplementary data related to this article can be found online at http://dx.doi.org/10.1016/j.thorsurg.2013.10.006.

REFERENCES

1. Johnson SB. Tracheobronchial injury. Semin Thorac Cardiovasc Surg 2008;20:52–7.
2. Schneider T, Volz K, Dienemann H, et al. Incidence and treatment modalities of tracheobronchial injuries in Germany. Interact Cardiovasc Thorac Surg 2009; 8:571–6.
3. Huh J, Milliken JC, Chen JC. Management of tracheobronchial injuries following blunt and penetrating trauma. Am Surg 1997;63:896–9.
4. Kiser AC, O'Brien SM, Detterbeck FC. Blunt tracheobronchial injuries: treatment and outcomes. Ann Thorac Surg 2001;71:2059–65.
5. Bertelsen S, Howitz P. Injuries of the trachea and bronchi. Thorax 1972;27:188–94.
6. Gussack GS, Jurkovich GJ, Luterman A. Laryngotracheal trauma: a Protocol approach to a rare injury. Laryngoscope 1986;96:660–5.
7. Symbas PN, Justicz AG, Ricketts RR. Rupture of the airways from blunt trauma: treatment of complex Injuries. Ann Thorac Surg 1992;54:177–83.
8. Lee RB. Traumatic injury of the cervico-thoracic trachea and major bronchi. Chest Surg Clin N Am 1997;7:285–304.
9. Kummer C, Netto FS, Rizoli S, et al. A review of traumatic airway injuries: potential implications for airway assessment and management. Injury 2007; 38:27–33.
10. Inci I, Ozçelik C, Taçyildiz I, et al. Penetrating chest injuries: unusually high incidence of high-velocity gunshot wounds in civilian practice. World J Surg 1998;22:438–42.
11. Kirsh MM, Orringer MB, Behrendt DM, et al. Management of tracheobronchial disruption secondary to nonpenetrating trauma. Ann Thorac Surg 1976; 22(1):93–101.
12. Karmy-Jones R, Wood DE. Traumatic injury to the trachea and bronchus. Thorac Surg Clin 2007;17: 35–46.
13. Glazer ES, Meyerson SL. Delayed presentation and treatment of tracheobronchial injuries due to blunt trauma. J Surg Educ 2008;65:302–8.
14. Farzanegan R, Alijanipour P, Akbarshahi H, et al. Major airways trauma, management and long term results. Ann Thorac Cardiovasc Surg 2011;17:544–51.
15. Chen JD, Shanmuganathan K, Mirvis SE, et al. Using CT to diagnose tracheal rupture. AJR Am J Roentgenol 2001;176:1273–80.
16. Rossbach MM, Johnson SB, Gomez MA, et al. Management of major tracheobronchial injuries: a 28-year experience. Ann Thorac Surg 1998;65:182–6.
17. Trupka A, Waydhas C, Hallfeldt KK, et al. Value of thoracic computed tomography in the first assessment of severely injured patients with blunt chest trauma: results of a prospective study. J Trauma 1997;43:405–11.
18. Scaglione M, Romano S, Pinto A, et al. Acute tracheobronchial injuries: impact of imaging on diagnosis and management implications. Eur J Radiol 2006;59:336–43.
19. Koletsis E, Prokakis C, Baltayiannis N, et al. Surgical decision making in tracheobronchial injuries on the basis of clinical evidences and the injury's anatomical setting: a retrospective analysis. Injury 2012; 43:1437–41.
20. Mussi A, Ambrogi MC, Ribechini A, et al. Acute major airway injuries: clinical features and management. Eur J Cardiothorac Surg 2001;20:46–52.
21. Rathlev NK, Modzon R, Bracken ME. Evaluation and management of neck trauma. Emerg Med Clin North Am 2007;25:679–94.
22. Mayglothling J, Duane TM, Gibbs M, et al. Emergency tracheal intubation immediately following traumatic injury: an Eastern Association for the Surgery of Trauma Practice Management Guideline. J Trauma Acute Care Surg 2012;73:S333–40.
23. Gomez-Caro A, Ausin P, Moradiellos FJ, et al. Role of conservative medical management of tracheobronchial injuries. J Trauma 2006;61:1426–34.
24. Carretta A, Melloni G, Bandiera A, et al. Conservative and surgical treatment of acute posttraumatic

tracheobronchial injuries. World J Surg 2011;35: 2568–74.

25. Grillo HC, Zannini P, Michelassi F. Complications of tracheal reconstruction: incidence, treatment and prevention. J Thorac Cardiovasc Surg 1986;91:322–8.
26. Bölükbas A, Schirren J. Parenchyma sparing bronchial sleeve resections in trauma, benign and malign diseases. Thorac Cardiovasc Surg 2010;58:32–7.
27. Weiman DS, Walker WA, Brosnan KM, et al. Combined tracheal and esophageal trauma from gunshot wounds. South Med J 1996;89:208–11.
28. Danić D, Prgomet D, Milicić D, et al. War injuries to the head and neck. Mil Med 1998;163:117–9.
29. Angelillo-Mackinlay T. Transcervical repair of distal membranous tracheal laceration. Ann Thorac Surg 1995;59:531–2.
30. Conti M, Pougeoise M, Wurtz A, et al. Management of postintubation tracheal membrane rupture. Chest 2006;130:412–8.
31. Trottier SJ, Hazard PB, Sakabu SA, et al. Posterior tracheal wall perforation during percutaneous dilational tracheostomy: an investigation into its mechanism and prevention. Chest 1999;115:1383–9.
32. Minambres E, Buron J, Ballesteros MA, et al. Tracheal rupture after endotracheal intubation: a literature systematic review. Eur J Cardiothorac Surg 2009;95:1056–62.
33. Welter S, Krbek T, Halder R, et al. A new technique for complete intraluminal repair of iatrogenic posterior tracheal lacerations. Interact Cardiovasc Thorac Surg 2011;12:6–9.
34. Cardillo G, Carbone L, Carleo F, et al. Tracheal lacerations after endotracheal intubation: a proposed morphological classification to guide non-surgical treatment. Eur J Cardiothorac Surg 2010;37:581–7.
35. Venkataramanappa V, Boujoukos AJ, Sakai T. The diagnostic challenge of a tracheal tear with a double-lumen endobronchial tube: massive air leak developing from the mouth during mechanical ventilation. J Clin Anesth 2011;23:66–70.
36. Schneider T, Storz K, Dienemann H, et al. Management of iatrogenic tracheobronchial injuries: a retrospective analysis of 29 cases. Ann Thorac Surg 2007;83:1960–4.
37. Kouerinis I, Loutsidis A, Hountis P, et al. Treatment of iatrogenic injury of membranous trachea with intercostal muscle flap. Ann Thorac Surg 2004; 78:85–6.
38. Okada S, Ishimori S, Yamagata S, et al. Videobronchoscope-assisted repair of the membranous tracheal laceration during insertion of a tracheostomy tube after tracheostomy. J Thorac Cardiovasc Surg 2002;124:837–8.
39. Park K, Lee JG, Lee CY, et al. Transcervical intraluminal repair of posterior membranous tracheal laceration through semi-lateral transverse tracheotomy. J Thorac Cardiovasc Surg 2007;134:1597–8.
40. Carbognani P, Bobbio A, Cattelani L, et al. Management of postintubation membranous tracheal rupture. Ann Thorac Surg 2004;77:406–9.
41. Meyer M. Iatrogenic tracheobronchial lesions – a report on 13 cases. Thorac Cardiovasc Surg 2001; 49:115–9.
42. Sippel M, Putensen C, Hirner A, et al. Tracheal rupture after endotracheal intubation: experience with management in 13 cases. J Thorac Cardiovasc Surg 2006;54:51–6.
43. Yamamoto S, Endo S, Endo T, et al. Successful silicon stent for life-threatening tracheal wall laceration. Ann Thorac Cardiovasc Surg 2013;19:49–51.
44. Marchese R, Mercadante S, Paglino G, et al. Tracheal stent to repair tracheal laceration after double-lumen intubation. Ann Thorac Surg 2012; 94:1001–3.

Tracheomalacia

Christian Kugler[a,*], Franz Stanzel[b]

KEYWORDS

• Tracheomalacia • Airway collapse • Dynamic airway CT • Aortopexy • Tracheoplasty

KEY POINTS

- Tracheomalacia is characterized by excessive collapsibility of the trachea, typically during expiration.
- Dynamic airway CT as a modification of the standard protocol seems to be a promising tool for noninvasive diagnosis of airway malacia.
- Surgery should be considered in severe symptomatic disease, especially in localized and segmental forms. Surgical lateropexia, tracheal resection, and surgical external stabilization are options.
- Tracheoplasty seems to be the best choice for selected cases of adult malacia.
- Surgery in children is different, due to the different causes. The most commonly performed surgical method is aortopexy.

TRACHEOMALACIA IN GENERAL

Malacia of the trachea, or tracheomalacia, comprises different conditions of the trachea that have a common impact: the tracheal walls are in close proximity. However, this manifests in different ways and from different causes. Tracheomalacia is both a dynamic and a fixed state. In general, the trachea changes its shape physiologically during the breathing cycle, depending on the pressure impact. Normally, there are certain phases during which the tracheal walls converge. The dynamic form of tracheomalacia may lead to an almost complete airway obstruction during regular breathing because the tracheal lumen is reduced to a slit or it is impassable (**Fig. 1**). This effect is significantly enhanced by extreme breathing maneuvers, such as coughing or the Valsalva maneuver. Tracheomalacia can affect the trachea in its complete length, only in certain segments, or in multiple segments. In addition, tracheomalacia can extend to the mainstem bronchi (tracheobronchomalacia).

Tracheomalacia is generally caused by one of two mechanisms: altered structures of the tracheal wall (eg, alterations of the tissue architecture or the elastic tissue characteristics)[1,2] or acquired secondary factors (eg, external compression or chronic inflammatory response).[3]

CLASSIFICATION OF TRACHEOMALACIA

In the literature, there are different approaches that systematically classify tracheomalacia based on different perspectives.[4] It seems rational to differentiate between tracheomalacia in children and adults.[5] Approaches that considered the different forms of the trachea lead to the classifications of saber-sheath (**Fig. 2**) and crescent shape.[6]

In 2005, Carden and colleagues[7] proposed a classification for tracheomalacia in both children and adults based on comprehensive reviews that differentiated between primary congenital causes and secondary acquired causes (**Boxes 1** and **2**).

In general, the well-known classification systems for tracheomalacia are organized merely descriptively and by factors from which no systematic considerations for treatment can be derived. In 2007, Freitag and colleagues[8] created

[a] LungenClinic Grosshansdorf, Wöhrendamm 80, Großhansdorf 22927, Germany; [b] Lung Clinic Hemer, Theo-Funccius-Str. 1, Hemer 58675, Germany
* Corresponding author.
E-mail address: c.kugler@lungenclinic.de

Thorac Surg Clin 24 (2014) 51–58
http://dx.doi.org/10.1016/j.thorsurg.2013.09.003

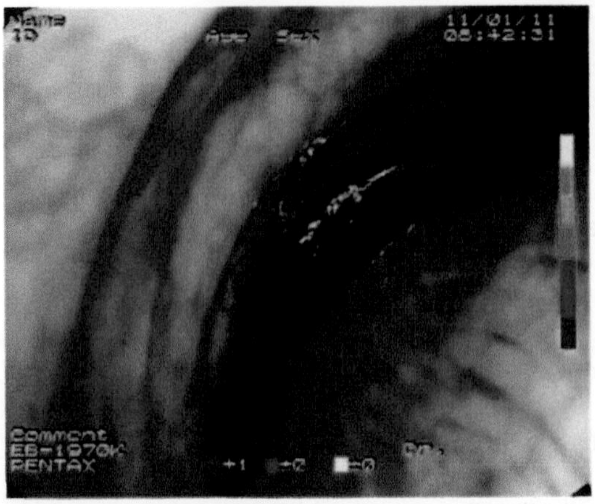

Fig. 1. Expiratory tracheal collapse in tracheomalacia due to chronic bronchitis.

a system for comparing therapeutic decisions and methods.

DIAGNOSIS OF AIRWAY MALACIA

Patients with airway malacia typically present with nonspecific chronic respiratory complaints, including dyspnea, cough, and recurrent infections. Thus, it is not possible to make the diagnosis of malacia based on clinical symptoms alone. Pulmonary function testing may provide supportive evidence of airway malacia but it is not diagnostic. Typically, there is a rapid decline of expiratory flow after a sharp peak that is associated with the collapse of central airways due to negative transmural pressure in the flow-volume curves. Conversely, the volume curve may be typically cropped due to stenosis. Despite sometimes typical findings, estimation of the severity cannot be made by pulmonary lung function testing.

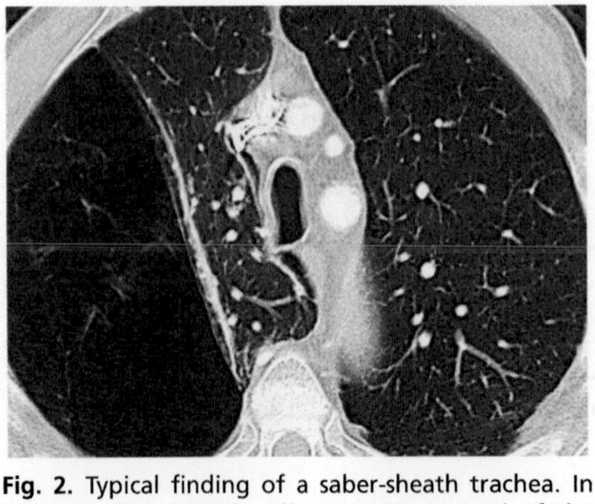

Fig. 2. Typical finding of a saber-sheath trachea. In this case, the lateral walls converge instead of the anterior and posterior tracheal walls.

Box 1
Classification of tracheomalacia in children

Congenital:

- Idiopathic
- Prematurity
- Congenital abnormalities of the cartilage
- Congenital syndromes associated with tracheomalacia
- Congenital anomalies associated with tracheomalacia

Acquired:

- Prolonged intubation
- Tracheotomy
- Severe tracheobronchitis
- External compression
  - Vascular
  - Cardiac
  - Skeletal
  - Tumors and cysts
- Infection
- Posttraumatic

Data from Carden KA, Boiselle PM, Waltz DA, et al. Tracheomalacia and tracheobronchomalacia in children and adults: an in-depth review. Chest 2005; 127:984–1005.

However, central airway collapse is not correlated with the degree of obstruction as assessed by forced expiratory volume in 1 second and central airway collapse may be found irrespective of the degree of expiratory flow limitation during quiet breathing.[9] There is no significant correlation between expiratory tracheal collapse and any pulmonary function measure. In a recent study, excessive expiratory tracheal collapse was observed in a subset of subjects with chronic obstructive pulmonary disease (COPD). However, the magnitude of collapse was independent of disease severity and did not correlate significantly with physiologic parameters.[10] There is a need for a standardized approach to evaluate airway malacia objectively in the patient with dyspnea refractory to traditional therapies.[11]

When pediatric pulmonologists expected to find airway malacia (based on symptoms, history, and lung function) before bronchoscopy, they were correct in 74% of the cases. In 52% of the airway malacia diagnoses, the diagnosis was not suspected before bronchoscopy.[12] Congenital malacia of the large airways is one of the few causes

Box 2
Classification of tracheomalacia in adults

Congenital:
- Genetic
- Idiopathic (Mounier-Kuhn syndrome) **(Fig. 3)**

Acquired:
- After intubation
- After tracheostomy
- Posttraumatic (chest trauma)
- After lung transplantation
- Emphysema
- Chronic infection or bronchitis
- Chronic inflammation
- External compression
  - Tumors (malignant, benign)
  - Cysts
  - Abscesses
  - Aortic aneurysm
- Vascular rings

Data from Carden KA, Boiselle PM, Waltz DA, et al. Tracheomalacia and tracheobronchomalacia in children and adults: an in-depth review. Chest 2005; 127:984–1005.

of irreversible airway obstruction in children, with symptoms varying from recurrent wheeze and recurrent lower airways infections to severe dyspnea and respiratory insufficiency. Children with mild airway malacia often present after the neonatal period with nonspecific symptoms such as rattling, wheeze, stridor, exercise intolerance, cough, recurrent lower airway infections, and airway obstruction.[12] Based on percentages between 23% and 57% of observed airway malacia in a pediatric bronchoscopic series, it was concluded that malacia of the central airways is more prevalent than previously thought, but general incidence data are lacking because of the lack of an objective definition or classification of airway malacia, and the lack of noninvasive diagnostic tests. Children with isolated airway malacia are easily misdiagnosed and treated for asthma instead.

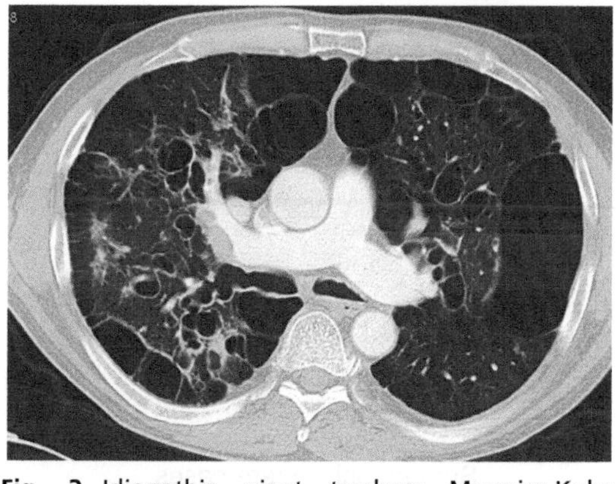

Fig. 3. Idiopathic giant trachea: Mounier-Kuhn syndrome.

Bronchoscopy is one of the methods for diagnosing airway malacia and is currently the gold standard. However, there is no widely used method for quantifying the degree of tracheal collapsibility other than specifying the extent of narrowing, which, in turn, depends on the pressure difference across the airway wall.[9] Most experts follow the rule that on bronchoscopy the presence of airway malacia is defined as greater than 50% expiratory reduction in the airway lumen. The severity of airway malacia is conventionally graded by the degree of airway collapse during forced expiration (intrathoracic malacia) or inspiration (extrathoracic malacia). Collapse less than 50% seems to be within normal limits, 50% to 75% is graded as mild, 75% to 90% as moderate, and 91% to 100% as severe malacia.[11]

During bronchoscopy, the collapse of the airways can be visualized directly and the extent and severity can be estimated. The diagnosis can be made and other causes for the symptoms excluded. Although most experts still agree that functional bronchoscopy is the gold standard for diagnosis, there are no standardized protocols guiding respiratory maneuvers and airway measurements during these procedures. Loring and colleagues[9] described a shape index based on images taken during bronchoscopy for more objective diagnosis of malacia.

Although bronchoscopy, especially with functional maneuvers, can reliably detect tracheomalacia, it may not be clinically feasible or desirable to perform this test in all patients who present with chronic cough and other nonspecific respiratory symptoms.[13] Tracheomalacia is widely considered an underdiagnosed condition because it cannot be detected with routine end-inspiratory imaging studies such as chest radiography and standard CT. An effective noninvasive tool makes more sense. Some advances in CT imaging afford the opportunity to diagnose tracheomalacia noninvasively using dynamic expiratory imaging (imaging during a forced exhalation).

Lee and colleagues[13] compared standard bronchoscopy for diagnosing malacia with a modified CT scan protocol, including imaging during two different phases of respiration: end-inspiratory and continuous dynamic expiratory. Helical scanning was performed in the craniocaudal dimension for both end-inspiratory and dynamic expiratory scans. The end-inspiratory scan is performed first. For the dynamic expiratory component, patients are instructed to take a deep breath in and to blow it out during the CT acquisition, which is coordinated to begin with the onset of the forced expiratory effort. A low-dose technique can be used for the dynamic expiratory sequence to minimize radiation exposure. Both end-inspiratory and dynamic expiratory images are assessed for evidence of malacia. The cross-sectional area of the airway lumen at the same level on end-inspiration determines the basis for calculation the degree of malacia. If the degree is greater than 50%, the diagnosis is malacia. The distribution of airway collapse can also be recorded. The sensitivity is 97% compared with the gold standard, bronchoscopy.[13]

Acquired airway malacia can cause central airway collapse in patients with COPD and may worsen airflow obstruction and symptoms. Tracheal collapsibility varies widely among these patients. Findings can be profound, such as tracheal narrowing during quiet breathing and substantial collapse only during forced exhalation. In one study, only 15% of subjects were not flow-limited during quiet breathing, 53% were flow-limited throughout exhalation, and 30% were flow-limited only during the latter part of the exhalation.[9] Subjects with flow limitation at rest showed greater tracheal narrowing than those without, but the severity of expiratory flow limitation was not closely related to tracheal collapsibility. On the other hand, some were flow-limited during quiet exhalation without central airway collapse. In tracheobronchomalacia, central airway collapse is not closely related to airflow obstruction, and expiratory flow limitation at rest often occurs in peripheral airways without central airway collapse.

There may be role for CT as a noninvasive, safe, and highly sensitive test to screen for the presence of malacia among patients with otherwise unexplained chronic respiratory symptoms who are at risk for this potentially treatable condition. Thus, bronchoscopy should be performed if clinical suspicion for malacia is high, despite a negative CT result.

THERAPY

Endoscopic Treatment

Current endoscopic treatments include techniques that splint the central airways, such as airway stents. In patients with severe symptomatic malacia, stenting may provide symptomatic relief through airway stabilization. Unfortunately, most reports of this approach are anecdotal. Ernst and colleagues[11] inserted silicone stents in 58 patients with severe disease. The main symptoms were dyspnea, cough, and/or chronic infections. There was symptomatic improvement in 45 out of 58 patients. However, there were also 49 complications reported, mostly stent obstructions, infections, and migrations.[11] Stenting is associated with a high number of short-term and long-term, but generally reversible, complications.[11,14] One problem with stenting in patients suffering from malacia is a high rate of migrations, especially of Dumon stents in subglottic stenosis. Fixation of stents may avoid migration. Other practitioners prefer Montgomery T-tubes in this situation. Generally, metal stents should be avoided in benign disease because of the much higher rate of reported complications and fractures. Stenting is also used for bridging for surgery or finding patients eligible for surgery. After stenting and improvement of symptoms, removal of the stent and surgery may be considered.

Surgical Treatment

Surgical treatment of tracheomalacia or tracheobronchomalacia is rarely performed. On the one hand, this may be necessary based on the type and extent of the medical situation. On the other hand, the advantage of such a procedure has to be justified. In most cases, localized causes or segmental manifestations are common subjects for surgery (**Fig. 4**).

It is always a question of an individual decision adapted to each situation with a defined

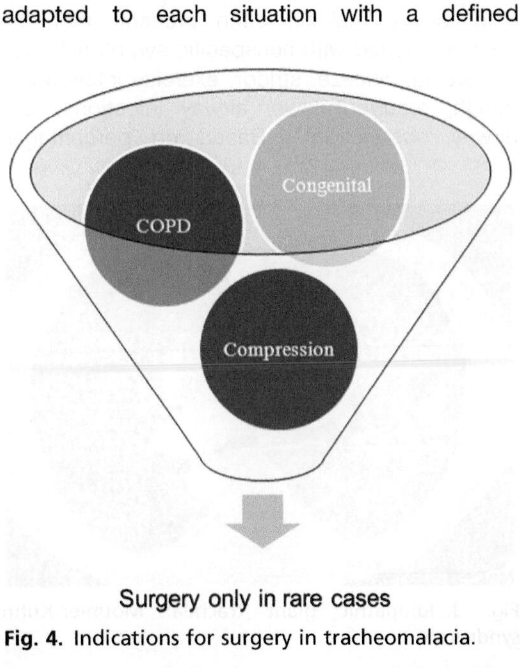

Fig. 4. Indications for surgery in tracheomalacia.

consideration of both risks and benefits. The correction of a static picture should never be the goal. Possible alternative treatments should be considered.

SURGICAL TREATMENT IN ADULTS

Extrinsic Compression

If the trachea is compromised externally due to chronic compression, the most common cause is compression by a goiter. This can be due to an enlarged thyroid in regular anatomic position, such as a goiter with intrathoracic expansion, or due to an ectopic thyroid with mediastinal localization (**Fig. 5**).[15]

In general, subtotal thyroid resection is sufficient for the treatment of tracheal stenosis. The likelihood of the separation of the trachea's external stabilization after a thyroid resection and of the emergence of a collapsed segment that requires an interventional procedure has not been evaluated consistently. It is reported in patients' collectives where this situation appears rarely but regularly.[16] There are also accounts that evaluate the improbability of such a problem. However, should such a situation occur, it is usually sufficient to bridge the time during which the trachea can harden in the operating area by mechanical ventilation. In the event of failure, there are additional possibilities for intervention:

- Insertion of a T-tube
- Tracheal stenting
- Different procedures of surgical lateropexia
- Tracheal resection
- Surgical external stabilization.

Tracheal resection is rarely needed, but may be performed if goiter resection for thyroid carcinoma is necessary and an infiltration of the trachea is present. In the past, external stabilization was established by implantation of bone grafts. Recently, porcelain or metallic clamps have been available, to which the trachea wall can be fixed.[17] In this case, it is important that the stitches are not completely transmural. It remains crucial that patients who are at potential risk are only operated on in a medical setting that has the corresponding emergency management available.

Occasionally, vascular malformation of the aortic arch and the supra-aortic vessels is first diagnosed in adulthood in terms of a vascular ring, (eg, a double aortic arch or an aortic arch located on the right side with modification of the supraclavicular vessels). These cases are often combined with tracheal compression. If the necessity for a correction arises, it is advisable to note that there is the possibility to evaluate the trachea endoluminally and, if necessary, to perform a procedure such as surgical fixation of the vessel. Even aneurysmatic changes of the aorta can lead to tracheobronchomalacia (**Fig. 6**), which may be corrected surgically.[18] Aside from the primary treatment of the vascular diseases, external stabilization procedures can be considered.[19]

After Tracheal Stoma or Intubation

Different possibilities have been discussed for the emergence of tracheomalacia after tracheal stoma or intubation.[3] On the one hand, ischemic necrosis of the cartilage may be responsible due to the pressure of the balloon cuff on the trachea wall. On the other hand, chronic inflammation reactions of the mucosa or a recurrent inflammation may be the cause. Thus, it is evident that more than one

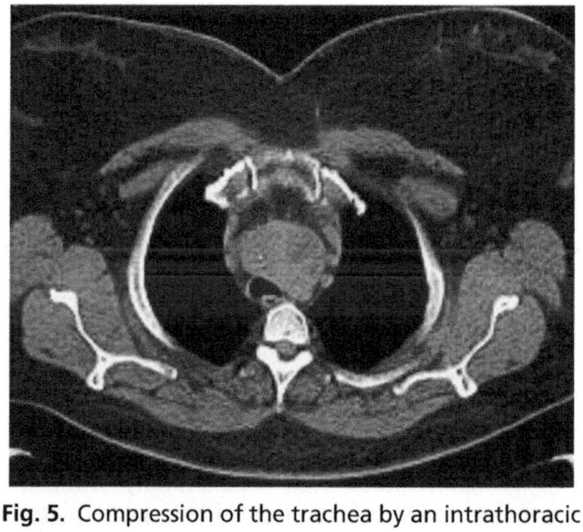

Fig. 5. Compression of the trachea by an intrathoracic goiter.

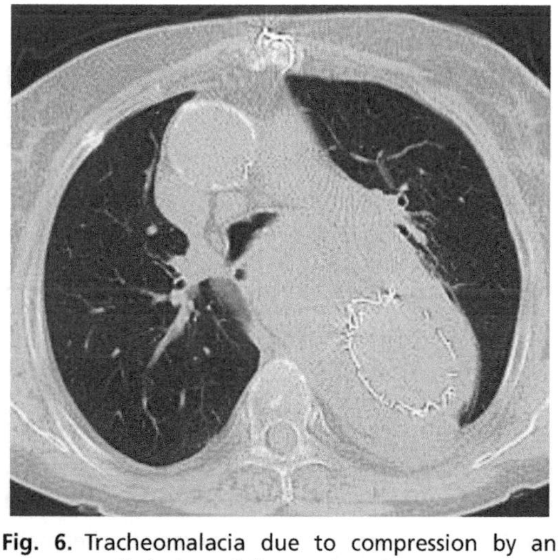

Fig. 6. Tracheomalacia due to compression by an aneurysmatic lesion of the aortic arch.

segment of the trachea may be compromised but, more commonly, two segments or the complete segment between the stoma of the tracheostomy and a distally located stenosis are affected. This is crucial for any surgical approach. If necessary for functional reasons, single segments with malacia are easy to remove via partial tracheal resection with end-to-end anastomosis (**Fig. 7**). Resection of a relevant segment leaving only heavily modified segments is unfavorable. Thus, the extent of the necessary complete resection may exceed the possible length compensation, despite all mobilization maneuvers. In this situation, the tracheal stoma may have to be preserved. In case of a stable structure on the front of the trachea wall in the region of the proximal resection line, the wall may possibly serve as a brace for a distal section of the trachea with structural damage by telescopic anastomosis.

In COPD

Tracheobronchomalacia in connection with COPD is characterized by changes that concern the complete tracheobronchial tree. It remains unclear whether this represents an expansion of the changes to the small airways or is a secondary effect of the primary disease.[20]

Concerning new surgical treatment approaches, however, it has to be considered that a peripheral airway collapse and the associated air trapping cannot be influenced by local treatment of the large airways.[13] Several symptoms, especially the retention of bronchial secretion, cough, dyspnea, and recurrent pulmonary infections, may be a result of an expiratory collapse of the large airways. The membranous wall approaches or even touches the ventral cartilaginous front wall of the trachea as a floppy membrane within the scope of the expiration. This mechanism depicts its own entity of a tracheal stenosis.[8]

In 1954, Herzog and Nissen,[21] and Nissen,[22] discussed this topic with the idea to influence the stiffness of the membranous wall. The concept was based on a tightening of the membranous wall, reinforced by bone grafts. Rainer and colleagues[23–25] seized this concept. After theoretical preparatory work, they introduced the surgical technique of membranous wall tracheoplasty and later published the long-term treatment results. Core elements of this surgical technique were the plication of the membranous wall, supported and reinforced by a strip of polypropylene mesh. The width of this strip is selected so that the back wall of the trachea obtains a normal dimension whereby the front wall of the trachea is remodeled generally similar to its original form. In addition to the edges of the tracheal back wall, the complete surface of the membranous wall is also fixed to the strip of mesh by multiple, nontransmurally applied sutures. Its aim is an in-growth of the tissue along the back wall of the trachea. The strip of mesh can extend above the level of the bifurcation to both main bronchi (**Fig. 8**).

The first results had problems concerning the reaction of the anatomic neighboring structures to the foreign material in terms of erosion in the trachea or the esophagus. In this respect, the surgical technique was revised by several investigators, especially concerning the materials used.[26] In addition to the polypropylene mesh, a Gore-Tex membrane (WL Gore & Associates, Inc, Flagstaff, AZ, USA) can also be used. Care has to be taken that only membranes that feature two different sides are used, and one side must be designed so that it can grow into the tissue. This side should be in contact with the membranous wall.

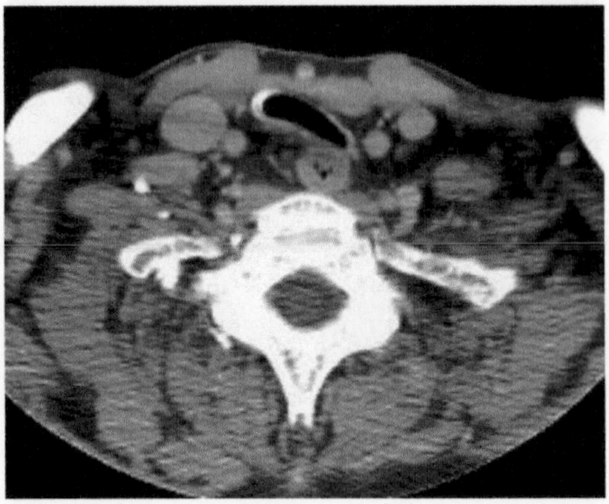

Fig. 7. A short segment of extrathoracic tracheomalacia; indication for surgical resection.

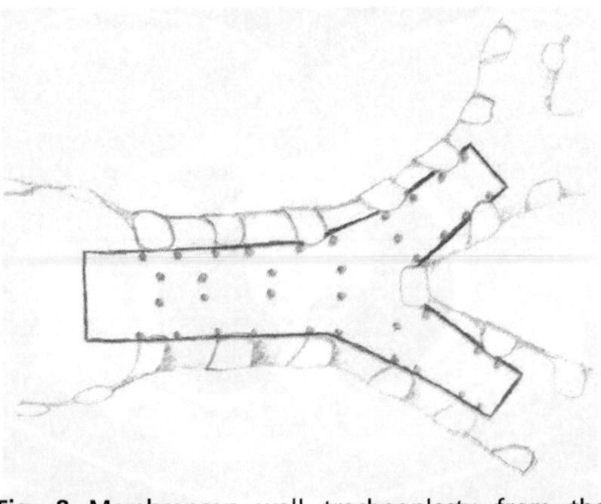

Fig. 8. Membranous wall tracheoplasty from the point of view of a right-sided posterolateral thoracotomy.

SURGICAL TREATMENT IN CHILDREN

Tracheomalacia in children is classified as idiopathic only in few cases. Most cases are associated with esophageal atresia or with an anomaly of the aortic arch or the supra-aortic vessels in terms of a vascular ring.[27–29] A significant amount of cases are caused by innominate artery compression. In some cases, arterial compression is not the only cause for tracheal stenosis but becomes relevant because of additional factors that create an increased pressure in the thoracic inlet, such as the herniation of a cervical thymus or congenital heart disease.[30] In most cases, if treatment becomes necessary, surgery is preferred to a stent application because of the latter's higher rate of morbidity and mortality.[31]

The most commonly performed surgical method is aortopexy. The aorta (possibly in combination with the proximal innominate artery) is fixed to the backside of the sternum (**Fig. 9**). Another surgical method that is sometimes considered is the transection of the innominate artery, especially in combination with severe chest deformity.[32]

Symptoms of tracheomalacia in infancy caused by vascular-related compression predominantly occur in the first 18 months of life. As the child grows (especially after the third year of life), the symptoms continually decrease and the morphologic causal situation improves. Therefore, a conservative treatment approach is usually justified. The respective symptoms are often heterogeneous; therefore, the indication for surgery is presented differently. Phases of apnea or multiple episodes of bronchopneumonia are also accepted indications for surgery, as are acute life-threatening events. Clinical and symptom-oriented diagnostics constitute the main basis for decision-making concerning treatment. MRI is the procedure of choice for evaluating compressive lesions of the trachea in children. A sole endoscopic result without any relevant clinical symptoms presents no indication for corrective measures. A reduction of the tracheal lumen by more than 70% is under consideration as a relevant endoscopic result.[33]

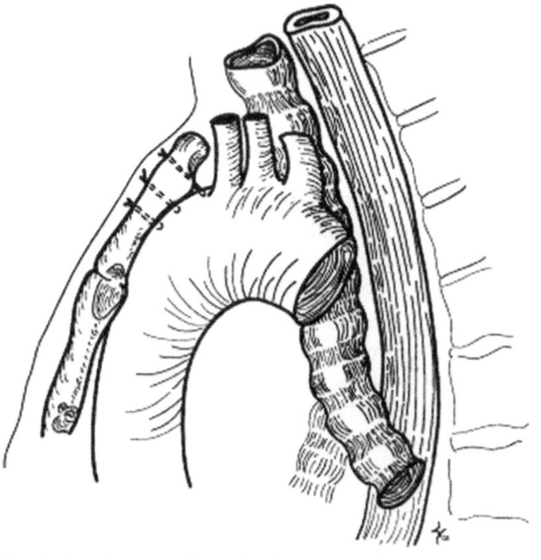

Fig. 9. Aortopexy. (*From* Weber TR, Keller MS, Fiore A. Aortic suspension (aortopexy) for severe tracheomalacia in infants and children. Am J Surg 2002;184:573–7; with permission.)

Good short-term as well as consistent long-term treatment results for surgical corrective measures have been described in both older and newer literature, especially for aortopexy.[27,34,35] Judged by the severity of the symptoms, the reported complication rates are tolerable. Aortopexy in children can also be performed thoracoscopically.[36] In rare cases, symptoms of vascular-related tracheomalacia can also persist into adulthood and, if appropriately diagnosed, may need treatment even then.

REFERENCES

1. Cox WL, Shaw RR. Congenital chondromalacia of the trachea. J Thorac Cardiovasc Surg 1965;49: 1033–9.
2. Wailoo M, Emery JL. Structure of the membranous trachea in children. Acta Anat 1980;106:254–61.
3. Feist JH, Johnson TH, Wilson RJ. Acquired tracheomalacia: etiology and differential diagnosis. Chest 1975;68:340–5.
4. Mair EA, Parsons DS. Pediatric tracheobronchomalacia and major airway collapse. Ann Otol Rhinol Laryngol 1992;101:300–9.
5. Masaoka A, Yamakawa Y, Niwa H, et al. Pediatric and adult tracheobronchomalacia. Eur J Cardiothorac Surg 1996;10:87–92.
6. Baxter JD, Dunbar JS. Tracheomalacia. Ann Otol Rhinol Laryngol 1963;72:1013–23.
7. Carden KA, Boiselle PM, Waltz DA, et al. Tracheomalacia and tracheobronchomalacia in children and adults: an in-depth review. Chest 2005;127: 984–1005.
8. Freitag L, Ernst A, Unger M, et al. A proposed classification system of central airway stenosis. Eur Respir J 2007;30:7–12.
9. Loring SH, O'Donnell CR, Feller-Kopman DJ, et al. Central airway mechanics and flow limitation in acquired tracheobronchomalacia. Chest 2007;131: 1118–24.
10. Boiselle PM, Michaud G, Roberts DH, et al. Dynamic expiratory tracheal collapse in COPD. Correlation with clinical and physiologic parameters. Chest 2012;142(6):1539–44.

11. Ernst A, Majid A, Feller-Kopman D, et al. Airway stabilization with silicone stents for treating adult tracheobronchomalacia. A prospective observational study. Chest 2007;132:609–16.
12. Boogaard R, Huijsmans SH, Pijnenburg MW, et al. Tracheomalacia and bronchomalacia in children: incidence and patient characteristics. Chest 2005; 128:3391–7.
13. Lee KS, Sun MR, Ernst A, et al. Comparison of dynamic expiratory CT with malacia: a pilot evaluation. Chest 2007;131:758–64.
14. Odell DA, Shah A, Gangadharan SP, et al. Airway stenting and tracheobronchoplasty improve respiratory symptoms in Mounier-Kuhn syndrome. Chest 2011;140(4):867–73.
15. White ML, Doherty GM, Gauger PG. Evidence-based surgical management of substernal goiter. World J Surg 2008;32(7):1285–300.
16. Agarwal A, Mishra AK, Gupta SK, et al. High incidence of tracheomalacia in longstanding goiters: experience from an endemic goiter region. World J Surg 2007;32(4):832–7.
17. Göbel G, Karaiskaki N, Gerlinger I, et al. Tracheal ceramic rings for tracheomalacia: a review after 17 years. Laryngoscope 2007;117(10):1741–4.
18. Pancini D, Mattioli S, Di Simone MP, et al. Syphilitic aortic aneurysm: a rare case of tracheomalacia. J Thorac Cardiovasc Surg 2003;126(3):900–2.
19. Tsubota N, Nakamura K, Nishiwaki M, et al. External support of collapsing tracheomalacia secondary to aortic aneurysm. Kobe J Med Sci 1987;33(5):197–204.
20. Kandaswamy C, Balasubramanian V. Review of adult tracheomalacia and its relationship with chronic obstructive pulmonary disease. Curr Opin Pulm Med 2009;15(2):113–9.
21. Herzog H, Nissen R. Relaxation an expiratory invagination of the membranous portion of the intrathoracic trachea and the main bronchi as cause of asphyxial attacks in bronchial asthma an the chronic asthmoid bronchitis of pulmonary emphysema. Schweiz Med Wochenschr 1954;84:217–21.
22. Nissen R. Tracheoplastik zur Beseitigung der Erschlaffung des membranousen Teils der intrathorakalen Luftröhre [abstract]. Schweiz Med Wochenschr 1954;84:219 [in German].
23. Rainer WG, Hutchinson D, Newby JP, et al. Major airway collapsibility in the pathogenesis of obstructive emphysema. J Thorac Cardiovasc Surg 1963; 46:559–67.
24. Rainer WG, Feiler EM, Kelble DL. Surgical technic of major airway support for pulmonary emphysema. Am J Surg 1965;110:786–9.
25. Rainer WG, Newby JP, Kelble DL. Long term results of tracheal support surgery for emphysema. Dis Chest 1968;53(6):765–72.
26. Wright CD. Tracheomalacia. Chest Surg Clin N Am 2003;13:349–57.
27. Torre M, Carlucci M, Speggiorin S, et al. Aortopexy for treatment of tracheomalacia in children: review of the literature. Ital J Pediatr 2012;38:62.
28. Rothenburg SS. Thoracoscopic repair of esophageal atresia and tracheoesophageal fistula in neonates, first decade's experience. Dis Esophagus 2013;26(4):359–64.
29. Triglia JM, Guys JM, Louis-Borrione C. Tracheomalacia caused by arterial compression in esophageal atresia. Ann Otol Rhinol Laryngol 1994; 103(7):516–21.
30. Mandell GA, McNicholas KW, Padman R, et al. Innominate artery compression of the trachea: relationship to cervical herniation of the normal thymus. Radiology 1994;190(1):131–5.
31. Valerie EP, Durant AC, Forte V, et al. A decade of using intraluminal tracheal/bronchial stents in the management of tracheomalacia and/or bronchomalacia: is it better than aortopexy? J Pediatr Surg 2005; 40(6):904–7.
32. Hisamatsu C, Okata Y, Zaima A, et al. Innominate artery transection for patients with severe chest deformity: optimal indication and timing. Pediatr Surg Int 2012;28(9):877–81.
33. Schuster T, Hecker WC, Ring-Mrozik E, et al. Tracheal compression by the brachiocephalic trunk in infants–surgical treatment of 30 cases. Z Kinderchir 1990;45(2):86–91.
34. Welz A, Reichart B, Weinhold C, et al. Innominate artery compression of the trachea in infancy and childhood: is surgical therapy justified? Thorac Cardiovasc Surg 1984;32(2):85–8.
35. Ley S, Loukanov T, Ley-Zaporazhan J, et al. Long-term outcomes after external tracheal stabilization due to congenital tracheal instability. Ann Thorac Surg 2010;89(3):918–25.
36. Perger L, Kim HB, Jaksic T, et al. Thoracoscopic aortopexy for treatment of tracheomalacia in infants and children. J Laparoendosc Adv Surg Tech A 2009; 19(Suppl 1):249–54.

Benign Stenosis of the Trachea

Erich Stoelben*, Aris Koryllos, Frank Beckers, Corinna Ludwig

KEYWORDS

• Trachea • Surgery • Stenosis • Bronchoscopy

KEY POINTS

- Benign stenosis of trachea results mainly from tracheotomy, ventilation, or trauma.
- The combination of a defect of the mucosa or the tracheal wall and infection produce secondary scar tissue healing with shrinkage of the tracheal lumen or instability of the tracheal wall.
- Injuries to the cricoid cartilage and the cricothyroid membrane increase the level of complexity for diagnosis and treatment.
- Clinical signs of stenosis, like stridor and dyspnea, appear when the lumen is obliterated by more than 50%; however, clinical signs and lung function testing are not very sensitive or specific for tracheal stenosis.
- Standard of treatment consists of resection of the pathologic segment of the trachea with end-to-end anastomosis.
- In case of involvement of the larynx, partial resections of the anterior cricoid cartilage or division of the larynx with tracheolaryngeal silicone stents is used.
- Short-term and long-term results are satisfying considering some technical recommendations.

HISTORY

Schüller, Gluck, and Zeller, as well as Küster, performed the first primary anastomoses of the trachea in animals and humans in the period from 1880 to 1890.[1,2] The low incidence of inflammation, trauma, and tumors of the trachea and the difficulties of ventilation during surgery limited further development in surgery of the trachea. In contrast, resection and anastomosis of the bronchus were introduced in thoracic surgery by Price Thomas in 1947[3] and widely used by Paulson and Shaw.[4]

Experimental surgery in animals and human cadavers in 1950 and 1960 with mobilization of the larynx and the pulmonary hilum (pericardial release) showed that up to half of the trachea could be resected. The basis for systematic tracheal surgery was created. In the meantime, intensive care medicine and mechanical ventilation found its use during the poliomyelitis epidemics and in cardiac surgery. The number of iatrogenic tracheal injuries and stenosis, due to high-pressure tube cuffs and an increasing incidence of tracheotomy, grew substantially, leading to the most important indications for tracheal surgery.[5]

CAUSES AND PATHOMECHANISMS OF BENIGN STENOSIS

Stenosis After Tracheotomy

Tracheotomy leads to a transmural defect of the ventral part of the cervical trachea. The tracheotomy wound is colonized by bacteria with local necrosis by mechanical alteration (**Fig. 1**). After removal of the tracheostomy tube, the defect is closed by the secondary scar tissue healing, which tends to contract. This process of healing results in an A-shaped stenosis of the trachea (**Figs. 2** and **3**). The severity of shrinkage depends on the extension of the defect, necrosis, and infection. The resulting stenosis is composed of contraction of the tracheostomy, instability, and granuloma of varying

The authors have nothing to disclose.
Thoracic Surgery, Lung Clinic, Hospital of Cologne, University of Witten/Herdecke, Ostmerheimer str. 200, Cologne 51109, Germany
* Corresponding author.
E-mail address: stoelbene@kliniken-koeln.de

Thorac Surg Clin 24 (2014) 59–65
http://dx.doi.org/10.1016/j.thorsurg.2013.09.001

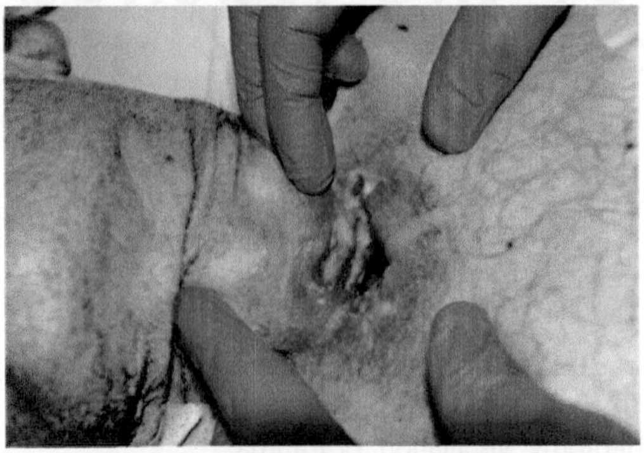

Fig. 1. Tracheostomy. Necrosis and chronic infection by mechanical alteration.

intensity. We do not understand how and why the local healing process ends up in either of the mechanical forms. When performing a tracheotomy, the surgeon should access the trachea at the level of the second to the fourth cartilage to avoid damage to the cricoid cartilage. Nevertheless, injury and infection of the cricoid and the cricothyroid membrane occurs and will increase the level of complexity for the diagnosis and treatment of this benign stenosis. Although the number of tracheotomies performed worldwide is high, the reports on late complications are rare, with differing results. The relevance of the technique of tracheotomy (Seldinger or surgical techniques) for late complications is unclear, as larger randomized studies have not been published.[6] The rate of stenosis after tracheotomy that have to be treated ranges from 1% to 20%.[7–13]

Cuff-Induced Stenosis

Low-volume, high-pressure cuffs of ventilation tubes induce circular necrosis of the tracheal mucosa.[14] Depending on the pressure, the duration of ischemia, and local infection, the underlying

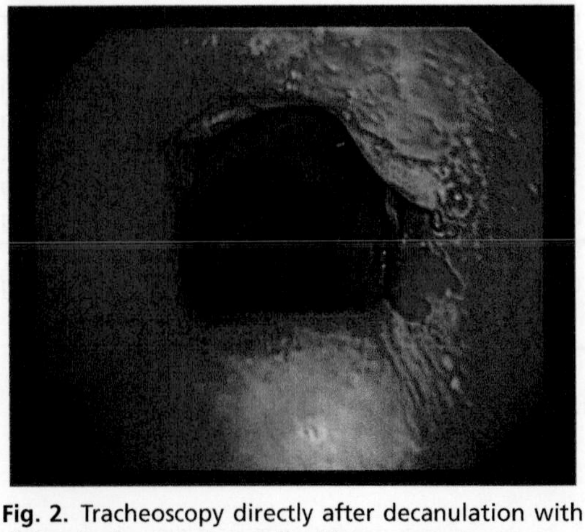

Fig. 2. Tracheoscopy directly after decanulation with defect in the anterior wall without stenosis.

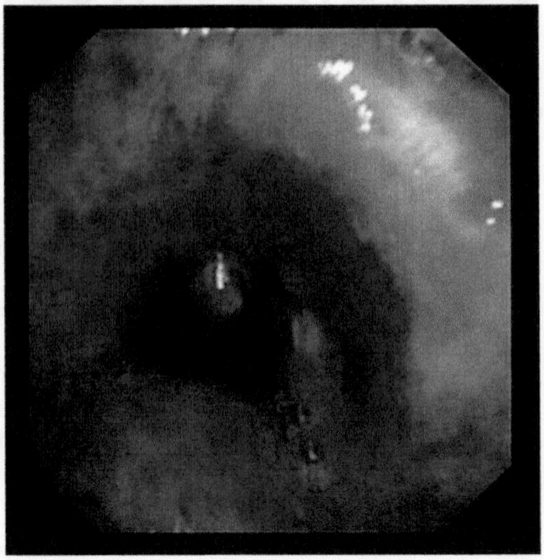

Fig. 3. Tracheoscopy 3 months later with stenosis by shrinkage and granulation tissue (same patient as in **Fig. 2**).

cartilages may be bare, necrotic, and destroyed. Mucosal defects without infection can be recovered from surrounding epithelium without relevant morbidity. Deeper destruction and infection of the tracheal wall leads to a ring of granulation tissue forming a sand-glass stenosis (**Figs. 4** and **5**). The malacia of the tracheal wall can be the main cause of stenosis and clinical symptoms. Similar to healing after tracheotomy, the reasons for different forms of stenosis remain unidentified. Cuff-induced stenosis appears in the middle part

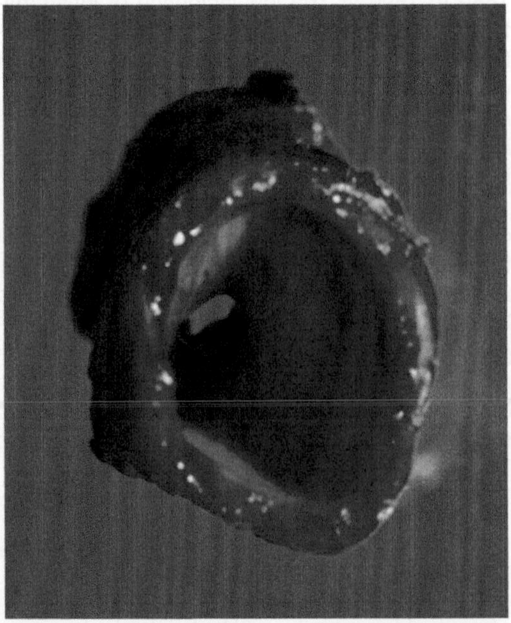

Fig. 4. Sand-glass stenosis after prolonged mechanical ventilation (cuff-induced circular necrosis).

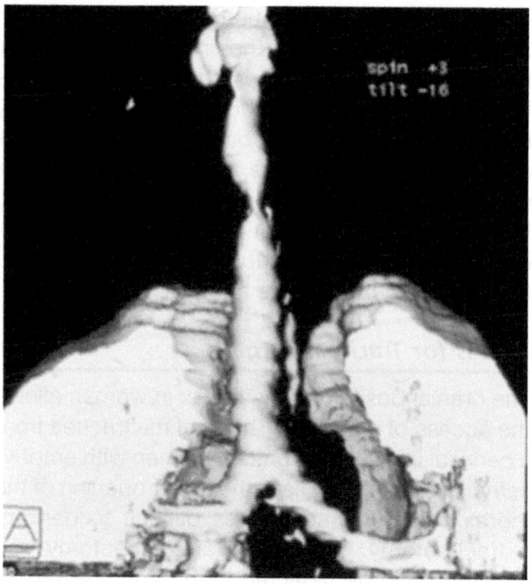

Fig. 5. Sand-glass stenosis, computed tomography reconstruction.

of the trachea. The introduction of low-pressure, high-volume cuffs make this kind of tracheal stenosis a rare disease.[8,15]

Idiopathic Inflammation and Stenosis

The disease occurs mainly in middle-aged women. The mucosa shows chronic inflammation with necrosis, granulocytic infiltration, and formation of scar tissue. The cartilage of the trachea, cricoid, and larynx is not affected. The inflammation and narrowing affects the subglottic trachea and can extend into the subglottic space of the larynx. Therefore, laryngotracheal operations with complex reconstruction are necessary when the stenosis is relevant.[16]

SYMPTOMS AND DIAGNOSTICS

Clinical Signs

Symptoms of tracheal obstruction can occur immediately after extubation or slowly over several years. Depending on the mechanism and the level of stenosis, a patient will show an inspiratory and/or expiratory stridor. The cough is ineffective and patient complaints include dyspnea caused by increased respiratory work load. Patients report a near normal function otherwise. In contrast, stair climbing or uphill walking leads to a rapid increase in the need for ventilation that cannot be satisfied. The resulting elevation of carbon dioxide induces a severe feeling of dyspnea and anxiety. At auscultation, one may find a sharp noise over the trachea, reflecting a turbulent air stream and the there is a short, barking cough.[17]

Lung Function Testing

Corresponding to the clinical symptoms, the spirometry reveals a fixed limitation of inspiratory or expiratory maximal flow rates. The other values normally used in thoracic surgery, such as forced expiratory volume in 1 second, underestimate the severity of the stenosis.[17,18]

The clinical signs and spirometry are not highly sensitive or specific for tracheal stenosis. Critically ill patients are often unable to communicate their respiratory problems. Furthermore, these patients cannot perform ergometric tests or cooperate in spirometry. Therefore, it is important to keep an eye on the patients after extubation and to consider tracheal stenosis when respiratory distress appears.

Bronchoscopy

Bronchoscopy is the standard procedure for the assessment of tracheal pathology. In spontaneously breathing patients, laryngeal function and anatomic localization of the main finding can be visualized. The severity of the stenosis can be estimated, although the subjective assessment misclassifies the objective loss of tracheal lumen.[18] The properties of the tracheal wall at the level of the stenosis can be described as granuloma, instable soft scar tissue, rigid scar tissue, or the combination of each of these. It is important not to oversee additional findings, such as anatomic variations or other sequelae of intensive care medicine, such as cuff-induced injury of the lower part of the trachea or other not-yet identified diseases, such as tracheobronchial tumors.[19] Furthermore, we recommend bronchoscopy before extubation of a patient with tracheotomy and before surgical closure of tracheostomies. It is important to detect injuries of the trachea and to avoid respiratory distress due to tracheal obliteration after extubation. Interventional bronchoscopy is a useful tool to treat patients with high-grade tracheal stenosis and respiratory decompensation. Dilatation, laser resection and sometimes stents (silicone) stabilize the respiratory function of the patient immediately and allow for planning of the surgical procedure.[19] There is little place for interventional bronchoscopy for definite treatment of tracheal stenosis apart from granulomas and webs.[20]

Computed Tomography Scan with Reconstruction

Helical computertomograms with high resolution and 3-dimensional reconstruction are able to visualize the trachea and deformations. Correlation with clinical symptoms is low. Mucus in the trachea and thin tracheal stenosis (webs) can lead to misinterpretation. Instability has to be investigated during inspiration and expiration. The accessory benefit of impressive radiographs in benign stenosis after bronchoscopy has not been definitely proven.[17,18,21,22]

Indication for treatment

Apart from the clinical symptoms of the patients, it is a challenge to define the indication for treatment objectively. The severity of stenosis corresponds to the drop of pressure over the stenotic segment in an experimental model with fixed stenosis. Using a flow rate of 30 L/min, the velocity of the air stream in up to 50% of obstructions does not exceed the velocity of the air stream in the glottis; 75%, 85%, and 90% of stenosis will increase the drop of pressure by a factor of 2, 5, and 10, respectively. Although this model does not meet all the criteria for tracheal stenosis in men (asymmetry, instability, varying velocity of the air stream), we should consider stenosis of more than 50% to be clinically relevant in consideration of the clinical symptoms of the patient.[23] This model concurs with clinical experience, as progressive stenosis by shrinkage can be missed until three-fourths of the lumen of the trachea is obliterated. If the process of obliteration proceeds, the patient will suffer from severe dyspnea and emergency treatment may be necessary. Murgu and Colt 2013 proposed the use of still bronchoscopic pictures combined with morphometric methods to measure the degree of stenosis objectively.

TREATMENT

Pretreatment by interventional bronchoscopy, emergency retracheotomy, and unsuccessful surgery may deteriorate the local situation by aggravating the stenosis or lengthening the damaged part of the trachea. The risk of complications after resection and anastomosis is increased by reoperation and depends on the length of resection.[24] For these reasons, we recommend avoiding any manipulation or surgery in nonexperienced hands. Different propositions for reconstruction of the trachea using artificial or organic material, transplants, or surrounding tissue have up until now not been able to achieve successful long-term therapy for these patients.[25]

Another important aspect of surgery in benign stenosis has not been systematically examined, although it might be relevant for postoperative success. Patients with a tracheotomy and long-term intensive care treatment tend to be colonized or infected by nosocomial germs, often with multi-resistant properties. Infection of the tracheotomy wound already contributes to the formation of tracheal stenosis.[8] At the time of surgery, local infection jeopardizes primary healing of the tracheal anastomosis and can lead to secondary healing with restenosis or insufficiency of the anastomosis.[26] Therefore, we recommend performing a microbiological culture and determining the resistance to antibiotics by diagnostic bronchoscopy before the operation to define the appropriate perioperative antibiotic treatment.[27]

Access for Tracheal Surgery

The cranial position of the larynx in women allows the access of about two-thirds of the trachea from a cervical incision. In contrast, in men with emphysema, the larynx can lie in the upper opening of the thorax, making it sometimes difficult to perform a tracheotomy. Stenosis after tracheotomy can nearly always be resected by a cervical incision. Cuff stenosis in the middle and lower part of the trachea needs a sternotomy or a right-sided thoracotomy. Planning the procedure and cooperation with the anesthetist is important for an uneventful operation. Intubation might be prepared by dilation of a tight stenosis before resection. Single-lumen tube and jet ventilation or intubation over the operation field are used for the transcervical and transthoracic approach.[28]

Trachea Resection with Anastomosis

Preparation should be performed strictly along the wall of the trachea to avoid damage to the laryngeal nerve. In patients with a history of trachea surgery, the identification of the brachiocephalic artery is important to avoid intraoperative bleeding. In most cases of benign stenosis, transverse resection and anastomosis of the healthy tracheal wall is possible without release maneuvers of the larynx or tracheal bifurcation. It is important to resect all necrotic and infected or destructed parts of the trachea to allow primary healing of the anastomosis. We use a single running suture technique with 3-0 or 4-0 polydioxanone and 2 needles. We commence with the suture of the posterior wall of the trachea (paries membranaceus) and progressively approximate the lateral wall from both sides to reduce the tension. After that, the patient's head is elevated by a pillow and the ends of the trachea are approximated as in a pulley block suspension (**Fig. 6**). The suture is finished in the middle of the anterior wall of the trachea. Suture techniques using monofilament, resorbable material with over-and-over stitches may have some advantages. Thread tension is well distributed and local necrosis under multiple knots is avoided. A monofilament running suture has the

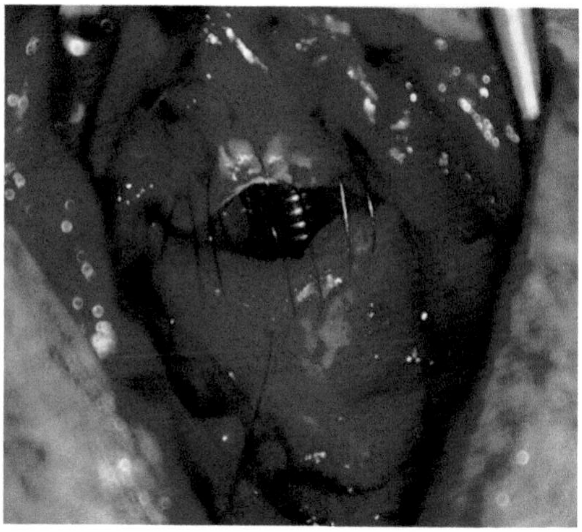

Fig. 6. Intraoperative view after end-to-end anastomosis with running suture just before closing the trachea.

advantage of reducing the quantity and the surface of suture material, which has a favorable effect on the inflammatory reaction in the tracheal wall.[29–31] There are currently limited data published about this important technical detail of tracheobronchial surgery.

In patients in whom the extent of the tracheal lesion is increased through interventional bronchoscopy or prior surgery, a tracheal resection of more than 4 cm could be necessary. The strain between the ends of the trachea reaches a level that reduces tissue perfusion and facilitates tearing out of the suture line. Beyond cervical flexion, the most important factor contributing to loss in tension is the laryngeal release, which can be used to mobilize the cranial part of the trachea. In contrast, the intrathoracic mobilization of the trachea and bifurcation should not provide any benefit to alleviate the anastomosis in cervical tracheal resection[32] due to the fixation of the intrathoracic trachea to the anterior surface of the esophagus. In our experience, the membrane between the distal trachea and pericardium can be transected by the cervical approach, which liberates the distal part of the trachea 1 to 2 cm upward.

EXTENSION INTO THE LARYNX

Trauma to the cricoid cartilage when performing tracheotomy leads to chronic infection with thickening of the perichondrium and the mucosa in the subglottic region. Other causes, such as cricothyroidotomy, idiopathic stenosis, trauma, postintubation, or Wegener disease, are rare. After tracheostomy with involvement of the cricoid, the anterior part of the cricoid cartilage has to be resected sparing the dorsal plate with the entrance of the recurrent nerves. In our experience of tracheal resections after tracheostomy, the anterior part of the cricoid has to be resected in a quarter of the patients. The distal end of the trachea has to be customized to fit well to the anastomotic line.

In the case of mucosal involvement of the posterior part of the cricoid, as in idiopathic or postintubation stenosis, the options range from dorsal mucosal flaps to splitting of the dorsal plate of the cricoid. In limited stenosis with thickening and cicatrization of the mucosa covering the dorsal plate of the cricoid, the defect after resection of the scar tissue is closed with a mucosa flap of the membranous wall of the trachea. In the case of extended stenosis of the larynx with circular cicatrization, the larynx can be widened by splitting the dorsal plate of the cricoid cartilage.[16,33] The more the surgeon accesses the larynx, the greater the risk of laryngeal edema and postoperative obstruction of the airway becomes. Therefore Montgomery T-tubes or more sophisticated tracheolaryngeal silicon stents are recommended as placeholders in complex laryngeal resections until healing is accomplished (up to 3 months) without obstruction.[34–37]

POSTOPERATIVE CARE

The patient is extubated as soon as possible. Intraoperative aspirated blood should be carefully removed before extubation. Recurrent nerve palsy can lead to inspiratory stridor and has to be distinguished from laryngeal edema by tracheoscopy. We emphasized previously the importance of preoperative microbiological investigations for effective antibiotic treatment. The use of corticosteroids and nonsteroidal anti-inflammatory drugs to treat edema can impair healing of the anastomosis and should be used only for a short period of a few days.[38,39] Aspiration is a common phenomenon after tracheal resection, especially in patients after laryngeal release and/or neurologic disorders. Assessment of speech and swallowing disorders before surgery may avoid postoperative complications in patients with neurologic disorders or prolonged illness. Bronchoscopy is indicated for diagnosis of edema, treatment of secretion retention, and control of healing of the anastomosis on the seventh postoperative day. The anastomosis is assessed by a standardized protocol that we use in tracheobronchial sleeve resections to decide whether the patients will leave the hospital or have to stay for further treatment.[40]

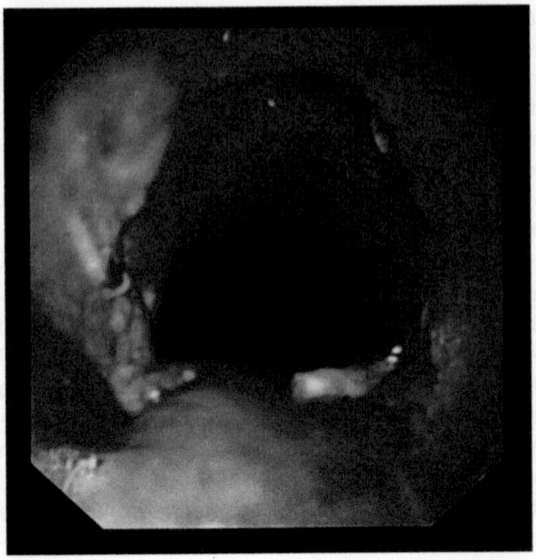

Fig. 7. Tracheoscopy 7 days after end-to-end anastomosis by running suture.

RESULTS

The aim of treatment is repair of the trachea with good respiratory function without further intervention. In contrast to interventional bronchoscopy of tracheal and tracheolaryngeal stenosis, resection and anastomosis of the trachea yields excellent results in more than 95% of patients (**Fig. 7**). The results depend on risk factors, such as repeated surgery, length of resection, or extended resection into the larynx, but the number of patients who will need definite treatment by tracheostomy will be fewer than 5%.[16,24,26,37,41] Therefore, surgical treatment of benign tracheal stenosis should be the treatment of choice. Cervical access and short operation times should allow surgery in nearly all patients independent of their comorbidities. The procedure ameliorates lung function with low complication rates in contrast to repeated bronchoscopic interventions in general anesthesia with high rates of intermittent complications, such as secretion retention and formation of granulation tissue.[19,42,43] No contraindications really exist for cervical tracheal resection in favor of interventional bronchoscopy.

REFERENCES

1. Grillo HC. Development of tracheal surgery: a historical review. Part 1: techniques of tracheal surgery. Ann Thorac Surg 2003;75:610–9.
2. Schüller M. Heilungsprocess der Trachealwunde. Deutsch Chir 1880;37:96–100.
3. Thomas CP. Conservative resection of the bronchial tree. J R Coll Surg Edinb 1956;1:169–86.
4. Paulson DL, Shaw RR. Bronchial anastomosis and bronchoplastic procedures in the interest of preservation of lung tissue. J Thorac Surg 1955;29:238–59.
5. Grillo HC. Development of tracheal surgery: a historical review. Part 2: treatment of tracheal diseases. Ann Thorac Surg 2003;75:1039–75.
6. Walz MK. Die Tracheotomie: Indikationen, Methoden, Risiken. Anaesthesist 2002;51:123–33.
7. Aboulker P, Lissac J, Saint-Paul O. De quelques accidents respiratoires dus au rétrécissement du calibre laryngotrachéal après trachéotomie. Acta Chir Belg 1960;6:553–61.
8. Sue RD, Susanto I. Long term complications of artificial airways. Clin Chest Med 2003;24:457–71.
9. Wagner F, Nasseri R, Laucke U, et al. Percutaneous dilatational tracheostomy: results and long-term outcome of critically ill patients following cardiac surgery. Thorac Cardiovasc Surg 1998;46:352–6.
10. Walz MK, Peitgen K, Thürauf N, et al. Percutaneous dilatational tracheotomy—early and long term outcome of 326 critically ill patients. Intensive Care Med 1998;24:685–90.
11. Melloni G, Muttini S, Gallioli G, et al. Surgical tracheostomy versus percutaneous tracheostomy. A prospective-randomized study with long-term follow up. J Cardiovasc Surg 2002;43:113–21.
12. Murphy DA, MacLean LD, Dobell AR. Tracheal stenosis as a complication of tracheotomy. Ann Thorac Surg 1966;2:44–51.
13. Florange W, Muller V, Forster E. Morphologie de la nécrose trachéale après trachéotomie et utilisation dúne prothèse respiratoire. Anesth Analg 1965;22:693–8.
14. Cooper JD, Grillo HC. The evolution of tracheal injury due to ventilatory assistance through cuffed tubes: a pathologic study. Ann Surg 1969;169:334–48.
15. Grillo HC. Postintubation stenosis. In: Grillo HC, editor. Surgery of the trachea and bronchi. Hamilton (Canada), London: Decker; 2004. p. 301–40.
16. Morcillo A, Wins R, Gómez-Caro A, et al. Single-staged laryngotracheal reconstruction for idiopathic tracheal stenosis. Ann Thorac Surg 2013;95:433–9.
17. Demedts M, Melissant C, Buyse B, et al. Correlation between functional, radiological and anatomical abnormalities in upper airway obstruction (UAO) due to tracheal stenosis. Acta Otorhinolaryngol Belg 1995;49:331–9.
18. Murgu S, Colt H. Subjective assessment using still bronchoscopic images misclassifies airway narrowing in laryngotracheal stenosis. Interact Cardiovasc Thorac Surg 2013;16:655–60.
19. Ernst A, Feller-Kopmann D, Becker HD, et al. Central airway obstruction. Am J Respir Crit Care Med 2004;169:1278–97.
20. Grillo HC. Stents and sense. Ann Thorac Surg 2000;70:1142.

21. Boiselle PM, Reynolds KF, Ernst A. Multiplanar and three-dimensional imaging of the central airways with multidetector CT. AJR Am J Roentgenol 2002; 179:301–8.
22. Glueckler T, Lang F, Bessler S, et al. 2D and 3D CT imaging correlated to rigid endoscopy in complex laryngotracheal stenosis. Eur Radiol 2001;11:50–4.
23. Brouns M, Jayaraju ST, Lacor C, et al. Tracheal stenosis: a flow dynamics study. J Appl Physiol 2007; 102:1178–84.
24. Wright CD, Grillo HC, Wain JC, et al. Anastomotic complications after tracheal resection: prognostic factors and management. J Thorac Cardiovasc Surg 2004;128:731–9.
25. Walles T. Tracheobronchial bio-engineering: biotechnology fulfilling unmet medical needs. Adv Drug Deliv Rev 2011;63:367–74.
26. Couraud L, Bruneteau A, Martigne C, et al. Prevention and treatment of complications and sequelae of tracheal resection anastomosis. Int Surg 1982; 67:235–9.
27. Wolter A, Ludwig C, Beckers F, et al. Influence of nosocomial infections on resection of tracheal stenosis after tracheotomy. Pneumologie 2012;66:7–11.
28. Hobai IA, Chhangani SV, Alfille PH. Anesthesia for tracheal resection and reconstruction. Anesthesiol Clin 2012;30:709–30.
29. Behrend M, Kluge E, Schuettler W, et al. Comparison of interrupted and continuous sutures for tracheal anastomoses in sheep. Eur J Surg 2002;168:101–6.
30. Friedman E, Perez-Atayde AR, Silvera M, et al. Growth of tracheal anastomoses in lambs. Comparison of PDS and Vicryl suture material and interrupted and continuous techniques. J Thorac Cardiovasc Surg 1990;100:188–93.
31. Scott RN, Faraci RP, Goodman DG, et al. The role of inflammation in bronchial stump healing. Ann Surg 1975;181:381–5.
32. Valesky A, Hohlbach G, Schildberg FW. Wertigkeit unterschiedlicher Maßnahmen zur Minderung der Anastomosenspannung nach Kontinuitätsresektion der Trachea. Langenbecks Arch Chir 1983;360: 59–69.
33. Grillo HC. Laryngotracheal reconstruction. In: Grillo HC, editor. Surgery of the trachea and bronchi. Hamilton (Canada), London: Decker; 2004. p. 549–68.
34. Conley JJ. Reconstruction of the subglottic air passage. Ann Otol Rhinol laryngol 1953;62:477–95.
35. Gerwat J, Bryce DP. The management of subglottic laryngeal stenosis by resection and direct anastomosis. Laryngoscope 1974;84:940–57.
36. Couraud L, Hafez A, Velly JF, et al. Current reconstructive management of subglottic stenosis of the larynx with reference to sixty consecutive treated cases. Thorac Cardiovasc Surg 1985;33:263–7.
37. Alshammari J, Monnier P. Airway stenting with the LT-Mold for severe glotto-subglottic stenosis or intractable aspiration: experience in 65 cases. Eur Arch Otorhinolaryngol 2012;269:2531–8.
38. Rendina EA, Venuta F, Ricci C. Effects of low-dose steroids on bronchial healing after sleeve resection. A clinical study. J Thorac Cardiovasc Surg 1992; 104:888–91.
39. Talasa DU, Naycib A, Atisc S, et al. The effects of corticosteroids and vitamin A on the healing of tracheal anastomoses. Int J Pediatr Otorhinolaryngol 2003;67:109–16.
40. Ludwig C, Stoelben E. A new classification of bronchial anastomosis after sleeve lobectomy. J Thorac Cardiovasc Surg 2012;144:808–12.
41. Grillo HC, Donahue DM, Mathisen DJ, et al. Postintubation tracheal stenosis; treatment and results. J Thorac Cardiovasc Surg 1995;109:486–93.
42. Schmidt B, Olze H, Borges A, et al. Endotracheal balloon dilatation and stent implantation in benign stenosis. Ann Thorac Surg 2001;71:1630–4.
43. Ryu YJ, Kim H, Yu CM, et al. Comparison of Natural and Dumon airway stents for the management of benign tracheobronchial stenosis. Respirology 2006;11:748–54.

Laryngotracheal Resection and Reconstruction

Ahmad Zeeshan, Frank Detterbeck*, Erich Hecker

KEYWORDS

• Laryngotracheal • Resection • Reconstruction • Subglottic Stenosis

KEY POINTS

- A thorough understanding of the extent of the stenosis and laryngotracheal anatomy is crucial before undertaking surgical repair.
- The posterior cricoid plate must be preserved to avoid recurrent laryngeal nerve injury.
- Careful attention to matching the geometry of the ends to be anastomosed is important to avoid gaps or weak points.
- The use of release maneuvers may be necessary if there is too much tension.
- High tracheal resection and reconstruction can be challenging and should not be underestimated by centers with little experience.

INTRODUCTION

The adult trachea is 10 to 12 cm long and consists of 16 to 20 horseshoe-shaped cartilages. High tracheal resections are uncommon and pose specific surgical challenges, and this is the focus of this article. Nonsurgical maneuvers are often used in preparation for surgery, but surgical treatment is often the final curative modality.

PRESENTATION AND DIAGNOSIS

The most common indication for high tracheal resection is symptomatic stenosis related to prolonged intubation or malignancy.[1,2] In 1 study,[3] 46 of 60 (77%) cases were for postintubation stenosis. Previous tracheostomy, fistulas, blunt trauma, and idiopathic causes account for the rest. The symptoms may include cough, stridor, dyspnea, or hemoptysis (malignancy). Fistulas may present as swallow-cough sign.

Clinical presentation is usually acute or chronic dyspnea. Acute presentation can be dramatic and may lead to a need for cardiopulmonary resuscitation. Chronic dyspnea may initially manifest with exertion only and then become persistent at rest. Sometimes, an acute flare is triggered by an upper respiratory tract infection. The trachea is usually narrowed up to 75% when acute symptoms are present in adults.[4]

Diagnostic modalities include rigid and flexible bronchoscopy and computed tomography. Direct laryngoscopy by an otolaryngologist is imperative in cases in which lesions extend into the glottis. Presence of enough subglottic space is required for a successful resection (**Fig. 1**).[1,5] Dilation, stenting, and T-tubes are used in selected cases in preparation for surgery.

ANESTHESIA FOR TRACHEAL RESECTION

Surgery for high tracheal resection requires specific anesthesia considerations. Muscle relaxants are usually avoided.[4] Frequent intraoperative communication between the surgeon and anesthesiologist is critical to the successful recovery of the patient. A small inflatable shoulder roll is usually used. Flexible and rigid bronchoscopy and dilation are used in the operating room just before the surgery in some cases to place an

Section of thoracic Surgery, Department of Surgery, Yale University, 330 Cedar Street, New Haven CT 06520-8062, USA
* Corresponding author.
E-mail address: frank.detterbeck@yale.edu

Thorac Surg Clin 24 (2014) 67–71
http://dx.doi.org/10.1016/j.thorsurg.2013.09.007

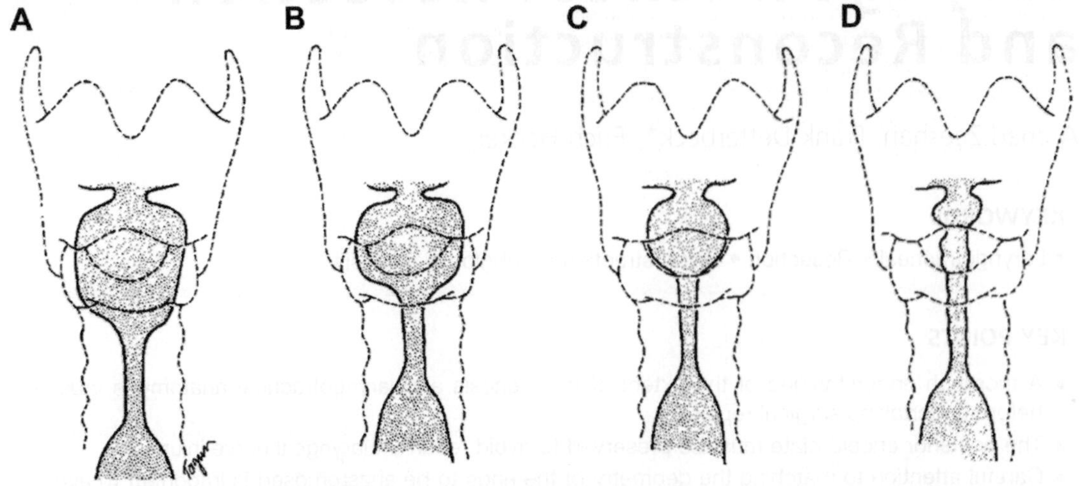

Fig. 1. Classification of upper airway stenosis. (*A*) High tracheal stenosis, easily treated by segmental resection and tracheotracheal anastomosis; (*B*) stenosis that reaches to the lower border of the cricoid cartilage; (*C*) stenosis of the lower subglottic larynx and upper trachea (the extent of the lesion involves the anterior portion of the cricoid cartilage); (*D*) stenosis that reaches to the glottis. There is no subglottic space to which an effective anastomosis can be made. (*From* Mathisen DJ. Subglottic stenosis. Operat Tech Thorac Cardiovasc Surg 1998;3(3):143; with permission.)

endotracheal tube, which is typically of a small caliber. A slow, deep induction while maintaining spontaneous breathing is often helpful.[1] Intraoperative jet ventilation can be used in selective cases.[6] A more detailed discussion is available in the article elsewhere in this issue by Wiedemann and Männle on Anesthesia and gas exchange in tracheal surgery.

SURGICAL TECHNIQUE

Tracheal resection and end-to-end anastomosis is the best surgical technique for the treatment of circumferential cervical tracheal stenosis. It is imperative that a tension-free anastomosis is created, otherwise, disruption of sutures occurs, leading to restenosis and other potentially life-threatening complications. If the gap between the 2 tracheal stumps cannot be closed without tension, tracheal release techniques must be used for a tension-free approximation.[7]

Incision and Exposure

A horizontal neck (collar) incision is used for initial exploration and is usually sufficient for high tracheal resections. A subplatysmal flap is raised, reaching the anterior border of the sternocleidomastoid muscles laterally. The sternohyoid and sternothyroid muscles are divided in the midline, and the thyroid gland isthmus is divided and ligated.[7] The anterior trachea is exposed in the midline from thyroid cartilage to suprasternal notch. In the case of a short trachea, the hilum should be exposed, typically through a median sternotomy.

Tracheal Resection

The length of stenosis is determined and the trachea is dissected circumferentially around it. Ideally, the area of circumferential dissection should not extend more than 1 cm above and below the area of resection to ensure adequate blood supply to the anastomosis. Thyroid arteries supply the cervical trachea, whereas bronchial arteries supply the mediastinal trachea. A vertical incision in the anterior trachea is made to evaluate the extent of narrowing.[1,8] If a stoma is present, the tracheal wall is divided vertically above and below the stoma.[7]

The trachea is sharply divided above and below the stenosis in normal tissue and limited to the area of stenosis to avoid ischemia of the stumps. Injury to the esophagus and recurrent laryngeal nerves (RLNs) could occur at this stage, if appropriate care is not taken. The endotracheal tube is pulled into the proximal trachea above the upper incision before the incision is made. For a high stenosis, it can be useful to tie a suture to the end of the endotracheal tube to facilitate subsequent retrieval. After complete resection of the affected segment, a second tube is introduced into the distal stump for ventilation.[7] An end-to-end tracheal anastomosis is constructed as described in the article elsewhere in this issue by Stoelben and colleagues on Benign stenosis of the trachea.

Usually, no more than 8 tracheal rings or 4 cm of tracheal length is excised to avoid anastomotic tension.[3] Tracheal release maneuvers are used if necessary to ensure a tension-free anastomosis. These maneuvers include suprahyoid and infrahyoid release and intrathoracic tracheal mobilization (carinal mobilization). Up to 6.4 cm of trachea can be excised with the use of release maneuvers.[9]

Cricotracheal Resection

Subglottic resections are challenging, because the cricoid cartilage is the only complete circumferential support for the airway and it has a close relationship to the RLN.[7] Segmental resection of cricoid and primary thyrotracheal anastomosis are accepted techniques.[1,5]

Circumferential dissection is not possible if the lesion extends well above the cricoid, because of the entry of the RLNs into the larynx.[1] The anterior and lateral walls of cricoid cartilage are removed, and the posterior portion is left in place (**Fig. 2**). The distal trachea is fashioned obliquely with an anterior prow to be anastomosed to the thyroid cartilage anteriorly and the residual cricoid posteriorly.

A submucosal flap may need to be removed posteriorly if there is mucosal thickening or scarring (**Fig. 3**).[1,5,7,8] The cricothyroid joints and entry of the RLNs limit the extent of resection superiorly. The RLNs should be identified on both sides before the resection of anterior cricoid cartilage.

Circumferential subglottic stenosis requires resection of the mucosa covering the posterior cricoid cartilage. The cartilage itself should be left intact, and dissection must stop just below the superior border of the cartilage, which is just below the arytenoid cartilages. When such a submucosal flap is removed from the posterior cricoid, a tailored flap of membranous trachea should be used to cover the denuded area (see **Fig. 3**).[1,5,8]

Previous laser surgery, irradiation, a long narrowed segment, and unusual locations may pose additional challenges to surgical resection.[1,10] The closer the stenosis is to the vocal cords, the more difficult it is to resect.[1] Laryngotracheal resections may involve very high lesions (Grillo type D, **Fig. 1**).[1]

Anastomotic technique

Two lateral traction sutures (2-0 silk) are placed to bring the 2 cut ends or the airway closer. These sutures are usually placed well above and 2 rings below the resection. Neck flexion is used as well at this point by deflating the shoulder bag. A 4-0 polyglactin or polydioxanone suture is used to anastomose the membranous trachea in a running or interrupted fashion. The knots are tied outside the trachea.[1,7] The traction sutures are then tied. At this stage, the endotracheal tube from the distal

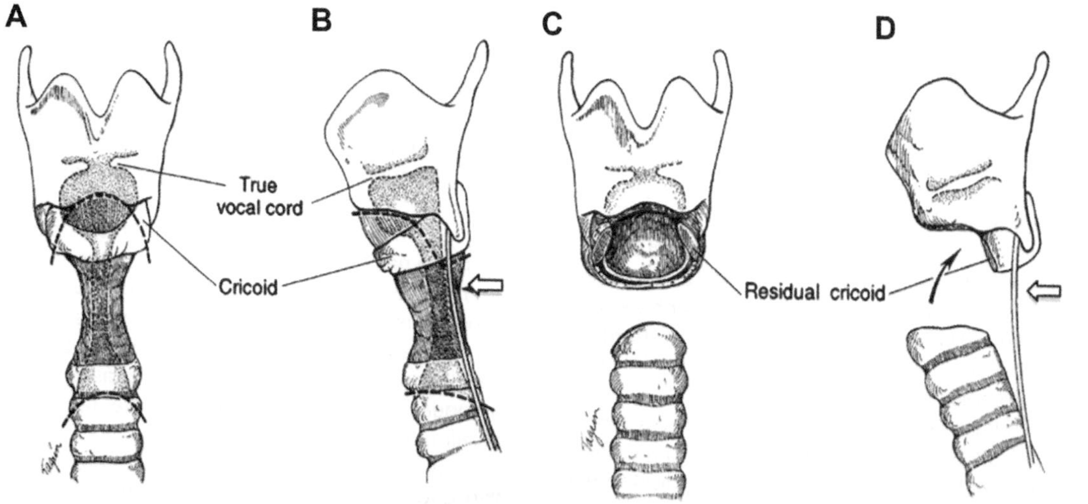

Fig. 2. High anterolateral stenosis. (*A, B*) The distal end of the lesion is identified and divided in an oblique fashion. The anterior (and lateral) portion of the cricoid cartilage is removed, leaving the posterior portion in place. This situation is caused by the proximity of the RLNs (*open arrow*). (*C, D*) The appropriately contoured distal tracheal end is anastomosed to the remaining cricoid and thyroid cartilage. Posterior sutures must go through the full thickness of the mucosal layer but may involve only a partial thickness of the cricoid cartilage; this makes placement easier and helps protect the RLNs (*open arrow*). (*From* Mathisen DJ. Subglottic stenosis. Operat Tech Thorac Cardiovasc Surg 1998;3(3):146; with permission.)

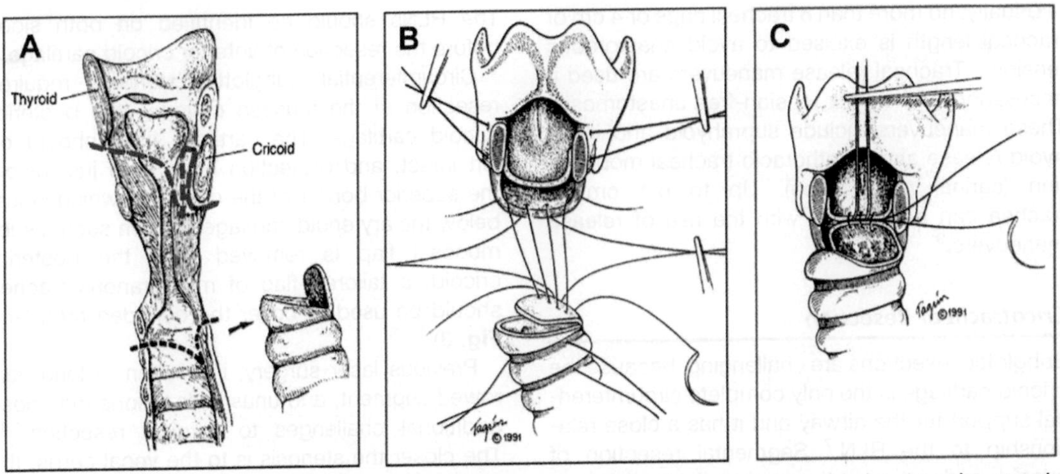

Fig. 3. Subglottic stenosis. (*A*) The line of mucosal division is carried up high on the cricoid plate in order to excise the involved mucosa and submucosa. Usually, the plane between mucosa and cartilage is dissected easily bluntly or with a scalpel, stopping just short of the superior border of the cricoid plate, which is immediately below the arytenoid cartilages. Subperichondrial resection of cartilage is not necessary. (*B*) Sutures are placed through the cartilaginous portion of the inferior margin of the cricoid plate and the outer portion of the membranous wall of the trachea below the proximal edge of the flap. These sutures fix the membranous wall posteriorly to the inferior edge of the cricoid plate and thus help to lay in the mucosal flap, which replaces the resected laryngeal mucosa. (*C*) Posterior mucosal sutures pass only through the full thickness of mucosa and submucosa of the posterior wall of the larynx and then through the full thickness of the leading edge of the membranous wall of the trachea. (*From* Mathisen DJ. Subglottic stenosis. Operat Tech Thorac Cardiovasc Surg 1998;3(3):149–150; with permission.)

stump is withdrawn and the orotracheal tube is advanced distal to the anastomosis.

When the posterior mucosa over the cricoid has been resected, the membranous trachea below the leading edge is first sewn to the lower border of the posterior cricoid cartilage (see **Fig. 3**).[1,5] Then, the posterior anastomosis is completed between the mucosa and submucosa of the posterior wall of the larynx and the edge of the prepared flap of the membranous tracheal wall.

Then, the anterolateral tracheotracheal anastomosis is performed in a continuous fashion. Sometimes, a second layer of reinforcing stitches is placed in the annular ligaments, 1 or 2 rings above and below the anastomosis. The tracheocricoid anastomosis is usually performed in an interrupted fashion. A muscle flap can be used to reinforce this anastomosis.

It is imperative that the anastomosis is tension free. Release incisions can be made to gain additional tracheal length. They include Montgomery suprahyoid release, hyoid release, pretracheal mobilization, and lateral finger dissection. These release incisions are described in more detail in the article elsewhere in this issue by Hecker and colleagues on Extended tracheal resections. The thyroid gland is usually approximated anterior to the anastomosis.

POSTOPERATIVE CARE

Usually, the endotracheal tube is removed in the operating room. If significant airway edema is noted intraoperatively, a small endotracheal tube is left in place. It is best to avoid leaving a tracheostomy tube in place through the incision on completion of the resection and reconstruction. Usually, after several days, the edema subsides and the patient can be extubated. Ventilation is typically not required after the patient recovers from anesthesia, because there is no injury to lung parenchyma. A chin stitch can be used to keep the neck in flexion and decrease the tension on the anastomosis, but most centers have abandoned this technique. Feeding tubes are usually not needed and patients can start oral intake on the second postoperative day. Occasionally, a laryngeal release may lead to some temporary impairment of swallowing.

However, it can be useful to mark an area on the skin and trachea for insertion of a tracheostomy tube should this subsequently be needed, because the altered anatomy may place the innominate artery or the anastomosis at risk without careful placement. If the patient continues to have difficulty breathing after a period of recovery with a small endotracheal tube on extubation in the operating room, the incision can be opened without extensive dissection. A small tracheostomy tube can then be placed below the anastomosis. It is usually difficult to place a small T-tube after a high resection, and it is best not to leave a foreign body in the subglottic area for a prolonged period in order to avoid restenosis in this area, which is difficult to treat.

MANAGEMENT OF COMPLICATIONS

Tracheal resection is a relatively safe procedure. Treatment failure occurs in less than 4% cases.[8] Postoperative bleeding may manifest as a cervical hematoma requiring a reoperation. Infections can manifest as mediastinitis and related sepsis. They are often difficult to treat. High resection endangers the RLN. Usually, patience allows this complication to resolve, but if it is permanent and unilateral, after several months, vocal cord medialization should be performed. An anastomotic leak or dehiscence is treated usually with a T-tube.[1] Suture granulomas require laser or bronchoscopic removal.[11] Recurrent stenosis occurs in about 10% of patients. Anastomotic infection, suture line tension, and subglottic resections are major predictors of recurrent stenosis.[12] Injury to the esophagus should be repaired primarily and augmented by a muscle flap.[7] Laryngotracheal resections, suprahyoid release, diabetes, reoperation, long segment resections, pediatric patients, and previous tracheostomy are associated with increased anastomotic complications.[10] The overall complication rate is approximately 18%.[11]

SUMMARY

High tracheal stenosis can be challenging, and there is little room for error. However, with experience, careful planning and meticulous technique, good results can be achieved. This procedure is best performed in experienced centers, which are also in the best position to manage complications; although rare mismanagement of these may result in an inability to salvage the airway or the larynx. However, most patients experience good outcomes with remarkable relief of dyspnea.

REFERENCES

1. Mathisen DJ. Subglottic stenosis. Operat Tech Thorac Cardiovasc Surg 1998;3(3):142–53.
2. Mutrie CJ, Eldaif SM, Rutledge CW, et al. Cervical tracheal resection: new lessons learned. Ann Thorac Surg 2011;91(4):1101–6.
3. Cordos I, Bolca C, Paleru C, et al. Sixty tracheal resections–single center experience. Interact Cardiovasc Thorac Surg 2009;8(1):62–5.
4. Mosafa BE, Chaouch-Mberek C, Halafi AE. Tracheal stenosis: diagnosis and treatment. Cairo (Egypt): Ain Shams University; 2012.
5. Grillo HC. Primary reconstruction of airway after resection of subglottic laryngeal and upper tracheal stenosis. Ann Thorac Surg 1982;33(1):3–18.
6. Wilkey BJ, Alfille P, Weitzel NS, et al. Anesthesia for tracheobronchial surgery. Semin Cardiothorac Vasc Anesth 2012;16(4):209–19.
7. Gavilan J, Toledano A, Cerdeira MA, et al. Tracheal resection and anastomosis. Operat Tech Otolaryngol Head Neck Surg 1997;8(3):122–9.
8. Grillo HC, Mathisen DJ, Wain JC. Laryngotracheal resection and reconstruction for subglottic stenosis. Ann Thorac Surg 1992;53(1):54–63.
9. Grillo HC, Mathisen DJ, Ashiku SK, et al. Successful treatment of idiopathic laryngotracheal stenosis by resection and primary anastomosis. Ann Otol Rhinol Laryngol 2003;112(9 Pt 1):798–800.
10. Wright CD, Grillo HC, Wain JC, et al. Anastomotic complications after tracheal resection: prognostic factors and management. J Thorac Cardiovasc Surg 2004;128(5):731–9.
11. Naeimi M, Naghibzadeh M, Mokhtari N, et al. Surgical treatment for patients with tracheal and subglottic stenosis. Med J Islam Repub Iran 2009;23(3):132–8.
12. Abbasidezfouli A, Akbarian E, Shadmehr MB, et al. The etiological factors of recurrence after tracheal resection and reconstruction in post-intubation stenosis. Interact Cardiovasc Thorac Surg 2009;9(3):446–9.

Treatment Approaches to Primary Tracheal Cancer

Dirk Behringer[a], Stefan Könemann[b], Erich Hecker[c,*]

KEYWORDS

• Tracheal cancer • Treatment • Radiotherapy • Chemotherapy • Combined modality

KEY POINTS

- A patient identified with tracheal cancer benefits most from evaluation by an experienced center.
- There should be an extensive effort to assess the possibility of a complete surgical resection as the most efficient treatment option for cure.
- Localized, nonoperable disease may still be controlled by combined modality using chemotherapy and concurrent radiation.

INTRODUCTION

Primary tracheal cancer represents a rare disease with a potentially curative therapeutic option, if localized. Standard of care with a curative intention should include complete surgical resection. Disease with locoregional extension that is not amenable to complete surgical resection requires combined therapy approaches in order to preserve the chance for long-term disease control. A specific therapeutic approach for locally advanced adenoid cystic carcinoma with a propensity for submucosal and perineural extension beyond the visible borders of the tumor is discussed separately. For palliative treatment of more extensive disease, systemic therapy has been used similar to treatment for lung or head and neck cancer.

To give patients access to potentially curative treatment, a diligent diagnostic workup, preferably in a center with expertise for tracheal tumors, is essential. Honings and colleagues[1] have recently suggested that in centers with experience, more than half of patients may be candidates for surgical resection, whereas in population-based studies, this treatment is applied to less than 25% of patients. Once the diagnosis has been established, treatment approaches should be discussed by a multidisciplinary board.

Surgery

Surgery has long been viewed as the primary curative treatment modality for malignant tracheal tumors. About 40% of these cancers are squamous cell cancers, with adenoid cystic tumors making up a similar proportion and other tumor types being rare.[2] Patients with squamous cancer typically present at a later age (60–70 years), are men (~90%), have a history of smoking, and have friable irregular endotracheal lesions. Adenoid cystic carcinomas occur in a broad age distribution (average ~45 years), have equal male/female distribution, and have more smooth endotracheal lesions.[1] Adenoid cystic carcinomas are discussed specifically later in this article.

The goal of surgical resection of a tracheal squamous carcinoma is an R0 resection. This goal can be achieved in about two-thirds of resections in

The authors have nothing to disclose.

[a] Department of Hematology, Oncology & Palliative Care, Thoraxzentrum Ruhrgebiet, Augusta Kliniken, Bergstr. 26, 44791 Bochum, Germany; [b] Thoraxzentrum Ruhrgebiet, Strahlentherapiezentrum Bochum, Bergstr. 25, 44791 Bochum, Germany; [c] Department of Thoracic Surgery, Thoraxzentrum Ruhrgebiet, Academic Hospital, University Duisburg-Essen, Hordeler Str. 7-9, 44651 Herne, Germany
* Corresponding author.
E-mail address: e.hecker@evk-herne.de

Thorac Surg Clin 24 (2014) 73–76
http://dx.doi.org/10.1016/j.thorsurg.2013.10.002
1547-4127/14/$ – see front matter

thoracic.theclinics.com

larger centers (**Table 1**). Most R1,2 resected patients have undergone adjuvant radiotherapy (RT). In one of the largest studies with a detailed analysis, a positive resection margin did not translate to worse survival (many received RT).[3]

The long-term survival rates in this group of patients seem to be reasonable (5-year survival of around 40% to 50%, 10-year survival of 20%–40%, see **Table 1**). The impact of nodal involvement, which is found in about 25% of surgical patients, is unclear, with larger studies showing either no difference or a nonsignificant trend to worse survival.[3,4]

A review of this experience points out several aspects of tracheal squamous carcinoma at the world's largest tracheal centers: (1) even at these centers, resection is performed in only a few patients per year, (2) many patients are able to undergo resection, (3) achieving a complete resection is difficult, (4) the operative mortality is low, and (5) 5-year and 10-year survival is reasonable. It is questionable whether lower-volume centers can achieve the same results.

RT

Indications for radiation include locoregional disease that is not amenable for complete surgical resection (contraindications to surgery include >50% of tracheal length involved by tumor, extensive locoregional tumor extension, poor patient performance status, and multiple positive nodal stations or distant metastasis, although a palliative resection may sometimes still be indicated in patients with adenoid cystic carcinoma).

In addition, sometimes, adjuvant RT is given after tumor resection with macroscopic or microscopic residual tumor and even after complete resection. Webb and colleagues[6] suggested adjuvant postoperative RT for most patients. The prognosis is better for patients who have adenoid cystic carcinoma than squamous cell carcinoma. The mean dose of adjuvant RT was 55 Gy; in some cases, adjuvant combined chemoradiation therapy was given. In patients presenting with distant metastases, chemotherapy has been used and was usually combined with local therapy, such as RT.

Radiation may be applied as an alternative to surgery in patients who do not qualify for surgery.

There are only scarce data on modern combined therapy approaches using high-precision radiation techniques such as image-guided RT (IGRT) and intensity-modulated RT (IMRT) or volumetric intensity-modulated arc therapy (VMAT) in combination with platinum-based chemotherapy, as has been established for locally advanced non–small cell lung cancer, which has resulted in long-term control of around 20%. Xie and colleagues[7] performed a matched-pair analysis of patients from the SEER (Surveillance Epidemiology and End Results) database with resectable and advanced tracheal malignancies, comparing patients who were treated with or without RT. Most patients had undergone a subtotal resection in both matched groups (only 5% in either arm underwent an R0 resection). Furthermore, there were no differences in age, gender, race, histology, disease extent (trachea only, trachea plus nodes, trachea plus regional organ extension). The investigators reported a significant overall survival benefit in the radiation group. Because most of the patients had squamous cell histology, this group was further analyzed, Overall survival was significantly better in patients undergoing surgery with RT versus surgery alone (5-year survival of 58% vs 7%; and a median survival of 91 months vs 12 months, respectively, but this study included few R0 resected patients). Among patients with squamous cell carcinoma treated without surgery, the survival was also better with radiation versus other (nonsurgical) treatments (4-year survival 41% vs 9%, with a median survival of 33 months vs 5 months, respectively). Although the retrospective nature of this analysis bears limitations, radiation in this setting apparently conveys a treatment advantage with acceptable toxicity.

For definitive therapy for tracheal cancer, a dose of 70 Gy in daily fractions of 1.8 to 2.0 Gy delivered

Table 1
Results of surgery for tracheal squamous carcinoma

Study	N	% of All Patients Seen	% Positive Nodes	% Positive Surgical Margin	% Operative Mortality	% 5-y Overall Survival	% 10-y Overall Survival
Regnard et al,[4] 1996	98	—	31	26	14	47	36
Gaissert et al,[3] 2004	90	66	27	40	4	39	18
Honings et al,[1] 2009	59	—	37	10	—	46	27
Grillo & Mathisen,[5] 1990	44	63	23	31	7	—	—

with external-beam RT is required, whereas 60 Gy is recommended in the adjuvant setting with microscopic residual disease.[1]

Combined Modality Approaches

Combined chemoradiation may be an option for inoperable patients with nonresectable localized disease. In 1 report, chemotherapy with cisplatinum, 5-fluorouracil and etoposide for 4 cycles was successfully combined with concurrent radiation of 60 Gy in 30 fractions in a patient with squamous cell carcinoma.[8]

These investigators suggested radiation doses of 60 Gy and higher to provide greater tumor control rates, but this might be associated with increased complication rates. To achieve a radiation dose increment, innovative high-precision radiation techniques like IGRT, IMRT, or VMAT offer the possibility of improving tumor control without increased side effects. These techniques offer the chance of highly conformal dose distribution to the target volumes, as shown in **Fig. 1**.

Recently, a similar approach has been applied in a young patient with unresectable localized disease and adenoid cystic carcinoma. The patient received 66 Gy of RT to the primary tumor volume. The radiation therapy was administered with concurrent weekly carboplatin (area under the curve, 2) and paclitaxel 50 mg/m^2 for 6 weeks.[9] The investigators concluded that in patients with unresectable disease, the short-term effectiveness of combined chemoradiotherapy suggests that a curative approach is justifiable in tracheal adenoid cystic carcinoma.

At our institution, we prefer a combination of cisplatinum (80 mg/m^2 on days 1 and 28) and vinorelbine (12.5 mg/m^2; days 1, 8, and 15) and concurrent radiation of 60 Gy or more, followed by an additional 2 cycles of the same chemotherapy (vinorelbine 25 mg/m^2; days 1, 8, and 15).

Specific Approach for Locally Advanced Cystic Adenocarcinoma

Adenoid cystic carcinoma has a propensity for submucosal and perineural extension beyond the visible borders of the tumor.[4,5,10,11] In locally advanced disease, the surgeon must frequently sacrifice complete resection of an adenoid cystic tumor to safely accomplish tracheal reconstruction, although this violates a basic surgical oncologic principle. Surgical resection margins are histologically positive in 40% to 50% of patients undergoing adenoid cystic carcinoma resection.[4,5,11,12] A nonsignificant trend toward poorer survival after incomplete resection has been reported in the larger studies (10-year survival, 64% and 69% for R0 vs 30% and 45% for R1,2 patients).[4,11] In addition, the incidence of suture line recurrence is low ($\leq$10%) in all patients undergoing resection of an adenoid cystic carcinoma (usually with adjuvant RT).[4,5,11] Survival after resection of adenoid cystic carcinoma is good, with 5-year and 10-year survival of 75% and 55%. Two studies did not find a survival difference between patients

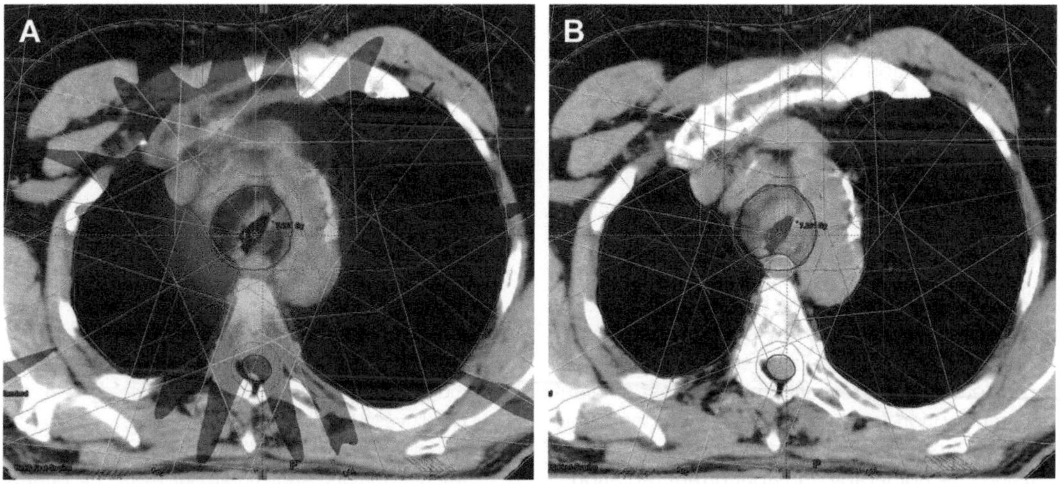

Fig. 1. Dose distribution of IMRT. The planning target volume (*red line*) is covered by the dose, as described earlier. Low-dose areas are painted blue, medium-dose areas green, and high-dose areas red (*A*). Maximal dose constraint is given to the organs at risk, such as lung, spinal cord, and esophagus. In (*B*), only the high-dose area, which is covering the planning target volume is colored (*blue and green*). With this high-precision radiation technique, dose reduction of lung, spinal cord (*blue*) and parts of the esophagus (*yellow*) was performed to reduce the potential side effect of these organs.

with or without node involvement.[4,11] It is important to have long follow-up of patients with these tumors, because these neoplasms typically show indolent growth. This characteristic is shown by the frequent finding of a long period (average, 1–2 years) of symptoms before a diagnosis is made[4,11,12] and survival of several patients for 5 to 16 years, even after the appearance of distant metastases.[10,11] Several investigators have reported late recurrences, appearing up to 27 years after the original resection.[5,13] Most patients, who underwent resection for adenoid cystic carcinoma, also received RT, especially if there was a positive margin or nodal involvement.[4,5,10,11] It is possible that the addition of RT has contributed to the good survival rate of these patients after resection. Although the 2 largest series found no survival advantage with adjuvant RT, the studies had insufficient power to show a modest survival advantage.[4,11] All of the centers with experience in treating this disease recommend RT for all patients, in the belief that this decreases the rate of recurrence.[4,5,10,11,14]

Systemic Palliative Chemotherapy

To the best of our knowledge, there are neither systematic reviews nor case reports on systemic palliative therapy in advanced tracheal cancer.

We choose chemotherapy regimens according to histologic subtype, similar to the practice with non–small cell lung cancer: combinations of platinum and vinorelbine or paclitaxel for squamous cell cancer and pemetrexed or gemcitabine in adenocarcinoma. In addition, we recommend molecular testing for activating somatic mutations of the epidermal growth receptor or EML-4-ALK, an activating mutation of echinoderm microtubule-associated proteinlike 4 fusing with the kinase domain of anaplastic lymphoma kinase, because these open additional therapeutic options with tyrosine kinase inhibitors.

SUMMARY

A patient identified with tracheal cancer benefits most from evaluation by an experienced center and an extensive effort to assess the possibility of a complete surgical resection as the most efficient treatment option for cure. Localized, nonoperable disease may still be controlled by combined modality using chemotherapy and concurrent radiation.

REFERENCES

1. Honings J, Gaissert HA, van der Heijden HF, et al. Clinical aspects and treatment of primary tracheal malignancies. Acta Otolaryngol 2010;130:763–72.
2. Gaissert HA, Honings J, Gokhale M. Treatment of tracheal tumors. Semin Thorac Cardiovasc Surg 2009;21(3):290–5.
3. Gaissert HA, Grillo HC, Shadmehr MB, et al. Long-term survival after resection of primary adenoid cystic and squamous cell carcinoma of the trachea and carina. Ann Thorac Surg 2004;78:1889–97.
4. Régnard JF, Fourquier P, Levasseur P, for The French Society of Cardiovascular Surgery. Results and prognostic factors in resections of primary tracheal tumors: a multicenter retrospective study. J Thorac Cardiovasc Surg 1996;111(4):808–14.
5. Grillo HC, Mathisen DJ. Primary tracheal tumors: treatment and results. Ann Thorac Surg 1990;49: 69–77.
6. Webb BD, Walsh GL, Roberts DB, et al. Primary tracheal malignant neoplasms. J Am Coll Surg 2006;202:237–46.
7. Xie L, Fan M, Sheets NC, et al. The use of radiation therapy appears to improve outcome in patients with malignant primary tracheal tumours: a SEER-based analysis. Int J Radiat Oncol Biol Phys 2012;84: 464–70.
8. Videtic MM, Campbell C, Vincent MD. Primary chemoradiation as definitive treatment for unresectable cancer of the trachea. Can Respir J 2003;10:143–4.
9. Allen AM, Rabin MS, Reilly JJ, et al. Unresectable adenoid cystic carcinoma of the trachea treated with chemoradiation. J Clin Oncol 2007; 25:5521–3.
10. Pearson FG, Todd TR, Cooper JD. Experience with primary neoplasms of the trachea and carina. J Thorac Cardiovasc Surg 1984;88:511–8.
11. Maziak DE, Todd TR, Keshavjee SH, et al. Adenoid cystic carcinoma of the airway: thirty-two-year experience. J Thorac Cardiovasc Surg 1996;112: 1522–32.
12. Azar T, Abdul-Karim FW, Tucker HM. Adenoid cystic carcinoma of the trachea. Laryngoscope 1998;108: 1297–300.
13. FG, Pearson. In discussion of Régnard F, Fourquier P, Levasseur P, et al. Results and prognostic factors in resections of primary tracheal tumors: a multicenter retrospective study. J Thorac Cardiovasc Surg 1996;111:808–14.
14. Refaely Y, Weissberg D. Surgical management of tracheal tumors. Ann Thorac Surg 1997;64:1429–33.

Carinal Resection and Sleeve Pneumonectomy

Walter Weder*, Ilhan Inci

KEYWORDS

• Sleeve pneumonectomy • Carina resection • Carinal pneumonectomy • Lung cancer

KEY POINTS

- Carinal resection and sleeve pneumonectomy are rare procedures and challenging issues in thoracic surgery.
- In spite of the knowledge of the technique, the incidence of postoperative complications is higher compared with standard resections.
- Adequate patient selection, improved anesthetic management and surgical technique, and better postoperative management might reduce the rate of postoperative morbidity and mortality.

INTRODUCTION

Neoplasms involving the main carina of the trachea constitute a major challenge for a thoracic surgeon in order to achieve a complete resection. The difficulty includes the dissection of the trachea and main bronchi, often together with other involved neighboring structures such as the vena cava superior, the resection of the carina, and the reconstruction of the airways.[1] The major difficulties are extended resections, in which the reanastomosed airways are under tension, and the surgeon has to judge beforehand how far he or she can go with his or her resection margins. Furthermore, there are different variations for reconstruction, and because the procedures are rare even in high-volume centers, few surgeons have relevant experience. Although the technique is well known and established, the incidence of relatively high postoperative complication rates makes this type of procedure more challenging, not only for the patient but also for the surgeon.

Recently, better patient selection, improved imaging techniques for surgical planning, improved anesthetic management and surgical technique, and better postoperative management have reduced the rate of postoperative morbidity and mortality.[2]

HISTORY

In 1950, Abbott reported on 4 patients who required right pneumonectomy with en bloc excision of the carina, lateral wall of the trachea, and part of the left main bronchus.[3] In 1959, Gibbon reported the first case of sleeve pneumonectomy.[4] He considered that the operation was palliative, and this patient died of local recurrence 6 months later. In 1966, Mathey and colleagues[5] reported the first European experience in 20 patients who underwent tracheal and tracheobronchial resection. They recommended circumferential resection with end-to-end anastomosis to reestablish airway continuity. Barclay and colleagues[6] reported their clinical experience with carina resection and primary reconstruction in 1957. In 1982, Grillo published his experience on carina resection in 36 patients and pioneered the modern era of the tracheal surgery.[7]

The authors have nothing to disclose.
Department of Thoracic Surgery, University Hospital, University of Zurich, Raemistrasse 100, Zurich 8091, Switzerland
* Corresponding author.
E-mail address: walter.weder@usz.ch

Thorac Surg Clin 24 (2014) 77–83
http://dx.doi.org/10.1016/j.thorsurg.2013.10.004
1547-4127/14/$ – see front matter

PATIENT SELECTION

Indications and Contraindications

Indications for a sleeve pneumonectomy (SP) or a carinal resection (CR) include nonsmall cell lung cancer, other airway tumors, and benign or inflammatory strictures.[8]

All patients who are candidates for SP or CR should be subjected to thorough medical screening, with special attention to cardiac and pulmonary function and coexisting medical diseases. Complete pulmonary function tests, arterial blood gas analysis, and quantitative ventilation/perfusion scans should be performed to help in the assessment of pre-and postoperative lung function.[9,10]

A predicted postoperative forced expiratory volume in the first second expiration (ppoFEV$_1$) value of 30% of predicted is suggested as the high-risk threshold for this parameter when included in an algorithm for assessment of pulmonary reserve before surgery.[11] Lung diffusion capacity for carbon monoxide (DLCO) should be routinely measured during preoperative evaluation of lung resection candidates regardless of whether the spirometric evaluation is abnormal.[11] A ppoDLCO value of 30% of predicted is suggested as the high-risk threshold for this parameter, when included in an algorithm for assessment of pulmonary reserve before surgery.[11]

Cardiac evaluation includes physical examination, electrocardiogram (ECG), and transthoracic echocardiography. In selected patients, cardiac single-photon emission computed tomography (SPECT) or coronary angiography could be needed to rule out occult coronary arterial problem.

The preoperative staging includes chest radiograph, CT scan of the chest and upper abdomen, positron emission tomography (PET) in case of a malignancy, and bronchoscopy. Bronchoscopy is the most important tool, as it usually helps mostly to identify a possible candidate for SP or CR. The degree of invasion should be documented by biopsies, and to take additional random biopsies 1 or 2 cm above the visible tumor is recommended.[2] These biopsies are important in order to achieve a complete resection, as a tension-free anastomosis is possible if the tumor does not extend beyond 2 cm of the lower trachea or beyond 1.5 cm of the opposite main bronchus.[2] For a tension-free reconstruction, a 4 cm distance between lower trachea and opposite bronchus is advocated.[12]

Preoperative irradiation more than 45 centigray is a relative contraindication to SP and even has been considered an absolute contraindication by some.[2]

Preoperative mediastinoscopy is indicated in patients with nonsmall cell lung cancer who are candidates for an SP or CR, because patients with lymph node metastases in the upper mediastinum have generally a poor prognosis.[1,2,10] Rea and colleagues[10] performed preoperative mediastinoscopy in PET scan-positive patients. Patients with histologically proven N2 disease underwent induction chemotherapy and were then reassessed with a repeat PET scan; responders or those with stable disease were scheduled for surgery. They did not recommend repeat mediastinoscopy in order to avoid excessive devascularization of the trachea.[10] de Perrot and colleagues[13] also reported the presence of metastatic mediastinal nodes to be a potential contraindication for surgery. They recommended performing mediastinoscopy routinely at the time of the planned CR to avoid the development of scar tissue along the trachea.

ANESTHESIA

During the operation, close cooperation between surgeon and anesthesiologist is required. Anesthetic techniques aim to maintain adequate anesthesia and gas exchange while providing a good surgical exposure.[2] Generally, anesthesia is maintained by either intubation of the remaining bronchus using a sterile endotracheal tube connected to sterile tubing passed off the anesthesiologist (cross-field ventilation) or jet ventilation (**Box 1**). In between intermittent apnea can be used to allow precise placement of the anastomotic sutures. As the far edge and posterior wall of the anastomosis are completed, the original endotracheal tube is advanced into the bronchus. Then anterior wall of the anastomosis can be reconstructed. High-frequency jet ventilation (HFJV) is another option. Because the tube used for ventilation is of small diameter, the surgical reconstruction is much easier to perform compared with a regular endobronchial tube. The use of extracorporeal membrane oxygenation (ECMO) to perform such complex operations has also been reported recently with good results.[14,15] It is restricted to situations in which single lung ventilation is not maintaining sufficient gas exchange.

Box 1
Anesthetic techniques

- Intermittent apnea
- Cross-field ventilation
- Extralong endotracheal tube
- HFJV (first choice of the authors)
- ECMO

SURGICAL TECHNIQUE

Anterolateral thoracotomy, posterolateral thoracotomy, or median sternotomy can be used to approach to carina. The preference of these approaches depends on the surgeon's experience.

Right Sleeve Pneumonectomy

Although most of the surgeons prefer posterolateral thoracotomy, the authors prefer an anterolateral thoracotomy. If the tumor is found to be resectable during the operation, the pulmonary artery and veins are encircled (if necessary intrapericardial) and divided with a vascular stapler. The azygos vein is divided with a stapler, and the vena cava superior is mobilized in order to obtain a good exposure of the carina. The distal trachea and the left main bronchus are exposed, mobilized, and encircled with tapes. It is important not to mobilize distal trachea too extensively in order to preserve the blood supply. The trachea is transected above the carina and the left main bronchus near its origin.[2] The distance of the resection line to the tumor should preferentially be 1 cm (**Fig. 1**A). Then the traction sutures are placed at the edge between the cartilaginous and membranous parts. At this moment, anesthesia is maintained either with cross-field ventilation or via HFJV (see **Fig. 1**B).

Although there are several ways to reconstruct the airway continuity, the authors prefer the technique in which running sutures are used for membranous part (see **Fig. 1**B), and interrupted sutures are used for the cartilaginous part (Polydiaxanone suture (PDS) 4/0, RB1 needle, Ethicon Inc., New Jersey). First a double armed PDS 4/0 suture at the contralateral edge is tied, and the membranous part is sutured in a running fashion beginning from the far edge. A few sunning stiches (3 or 4) are done at the cartilaginous part to reanastomose the far edge. After completing the membranous part, the stay suture on the near edge is tied. For the reconstruction of the rest of the cartilaginous part, interrupted sutures are inserted (see **Fig. 1**C). The sutures are tied after they all have been inserted (see **Fig. 1**D). Before tying the sutures, cross-field ventilation or jet ventilation is replaced with the original endotracheal tube. The

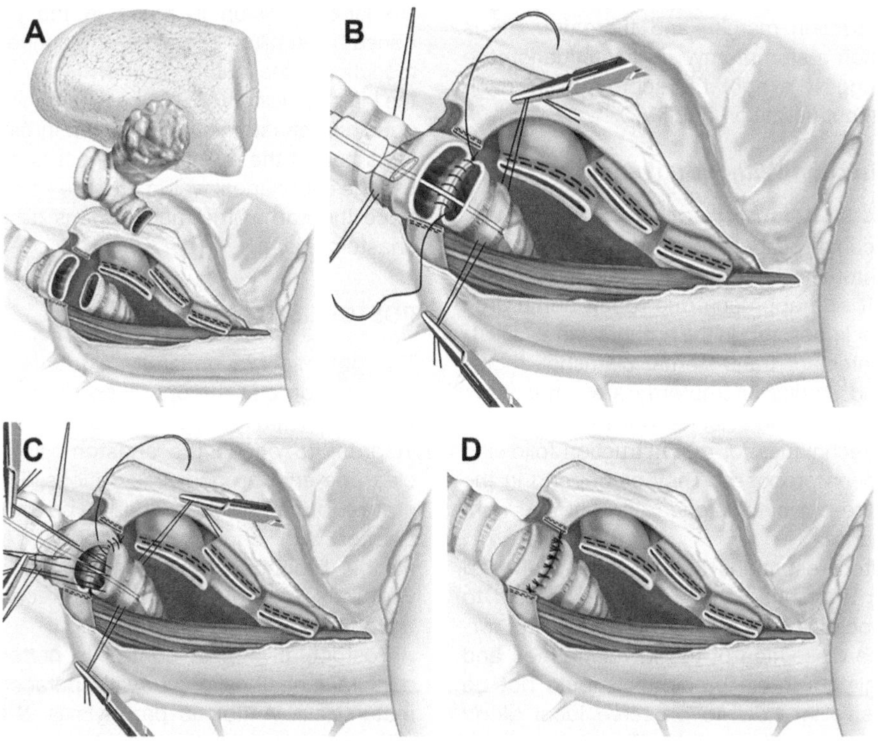

Fig. 1. (*A*) The pulmonary artery and veins are divided with a vascular stapler. The azygos vein is divided with a stapler, and the vena cava superior is mobilized in order to obtain a better exposure. The distal trachea and the left main bronchus are exposed, mobilized, and encircled with tapes. (*B*) First the stay suture at the contralateral edge is tied, and the membranous part is sutured in a running fashion beginning from the far edge. After completing the membranous part, the stay suture on the near edge is tied. (*C*) For the reconstruction of the cartilaginous part, the authors start from the far edge with an already knotted suture of this edge with 3 or 4 continuous stiches and then insert interrupted sutures. (*D*) The sutures are tied after they all have been inserted.

anastomosis is covered with a viable tissue, either with intercostal muscle flap or pericardial fat.[2] Then the anastomosis checked for air leaks under water following flexible bronchoscopy.

Left Sleeve Pneumonectomy

Left sleeve pneumonectomy is rarely performed. The reasons are that the left main bronchus is longer than the right main bronchus, and the left main bronchus usually invades the structures of the subaortic space.[16] A positive resection margin after a standard left pneumonectomy is the most common indication for left SP.

For a planned left SP, there are different approaches. It can be performed via median sternotomy,[2] hemi-clamshell incision or as suggested by Porhanov and colleagues[1] transection of the pulmonary artery and veins with video-assisted thoracoscopic surgery (VATS) and completion of the procedure via sternotomy.

For an unplanned left SP (eg, positive resection margin), SP can be performed during the same operation (1-stage procedure)[12,17,18] or later (2-stage procedure). For a 2-stage procedure, the pneumonectomy is completed, accepting a positive resection margin, and thereafter SP is done through a sternotomy.[2] In this situation the authors suggest a right thoracotomy approach with or without utilization of ECMO.

Carina Resection Without Pulmonary Resection

The most common approach for CR is right thoracotomy through the fourth or fifth intercostal space. Left side approach due to left aortic arch is difficult or impossible in the authors' view.[9] Bilateral submammary trans-sternal clamshell thoracotomy and median sternotomy are other ways to approach carina in selected patients.[19]

Various techniques for reconstruction following CR have been proposed. They all depend in the extent of the resected trachea and left and right main bronchus.[9]

For limited resections of the carina, left and right main bronchus can be reapproximated to form a neocarina.[8,9] For CR with neocarina formation, the dissection of the lower trachea and the contralateral main bronchus should not be too extensive in order to preserve local blood supply as much as possible. First the authors reconstruct the neocarina. For this, they insert the first stich between the cartilaginous and membranous portion of the 2 main bronchi. After knotting the cartilaginous part a running suture is done in the middle to reconstruct the "neocarina". Then the membranous part of the trachea is reconstructed with the membranous part of the bronchi with a running suture beginning from the far edge and coming to the near edge. The anterior wall (cartilaginous portion) is completed with interrupted sutures placed and tied at the end (**Fig. 2**). For CR with extensive airway resection, the trachea can be anastomosed end to end with either right or left main bronchus, with the contralateral bronchus reimplanted into the side of the trachea.[20]

SPECIAL TECHNICAL CONSIDERATIONS IN EXTENSIVE RESECTIONS

An important factor in technical failure after CR and CP is excessive tension at the anastomosis performed.[9] The easiest and well-known maneuver is flexion of the neck, which allows devolvement of trachea into the mediastinum.[9] The mobilization of the anterior pretracheal plane also provides some mobility to the trachea.[9]

A considerable reduction in anastomotic tension can be achieved by mobilization of the hilum using inferior hilar release on either side. Following the division of the inferior pulmonary ligament, a U-shaped incision is made in the pericardium beneath the hilum.[9] In case of planned extensive resections, the authors perform hilar release on the left side using VATS. In case of fragile membranous part anastomosis of if a gap in the membranous part of the anastomosis occurs, the authors use the esophageal wall in order to cover and reinforce the gap in the membranous portion of the anastomosis.

POSTOPERATIVE CARE

The patients are generally extubated following the procedure in the operating room. Before extubation, flexible bronchoscopy should be done in order to check the anastomosis again and clear the endobronchial secretions. The postoperative bronchorrehea should be preferentially treated with chest physiotherapy. A bedside flexible bronchoscopy is rarely needed. In severe cases, prophylactic mini-tracheotomy is advocated.[2,21]

Postoperative pain control is performed with epidural anesthesia and with paracetamol and metamizole. Antibiotic prophylaxis is performed with amoxicillin clavulanic acid at least 7 days.

Following CR and reconstruction, a heavy stitch between the chin and chest is recommended, avoiding excessive tension in the early postoperative period for 7 days; however, the authors do not use this technique and have had no complication at the airways.[9]

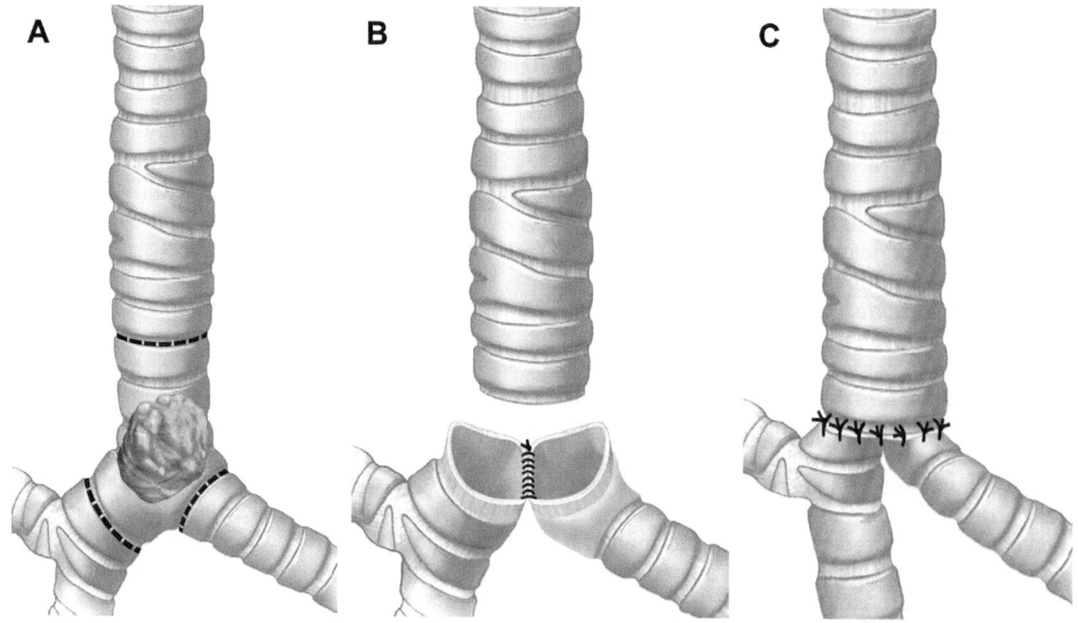

Fig. 2. (*A, B*) For carina resection with neocarina formation, the authors initially insert the first stich between the cartilaginous and membranous portion of the 2 main bronchi. After knotting the cartilaginous part a running suture is done in the middle to reconstruct the "neocarina". (*C*) Then the membranous part of the trachea is reconstructed with the membranous part of the bronchi with a running suture, beginning from the far edge and coming to the near edge. The anterior wall (cartilaginous portion) is completed with interrupted sutures placed and tied at the end.

MORBIDITY, MORTALITY, AND SURVIVAL

Acute respiratory distress syndrome (ARDS) is a life-threatening complication that occurs in up to 20% of SP cases and has a mortality rate of 50% to 100%.[10,13,22] Ventilator-induced injury and fluid overload during surgery are referred as the risk factors.[22–24] Porhanov and colleagues[1] reported the use of HFJV as a risk factor for development of ARDS, which occurred in 8 of 11 cases. Contrary to this observation, Rea and colleagues[10] reported only 2% ARDS cases in those managed with HFJV.

Anastomotic complications vary from granulation tissue, necrosis, mucosal sloughing, and microfistula to life-threatening dehiscence of the anastomosis.[10] According to Deslauriers and colleagues[2] broncho-pleural fistulas (BPF) are uncommon if the anastomosis is healthy and covered with a viable tissue. High-dose preoperative radiotherapy can increase the risk of BPF formation.[25] Jensik and colleagues[26] reported 6 BPF cases in their 34 patients. Five of those had preoperative radiotherapy. Airway resection limited to 4 cm, avoidance of bronchial devascularization, precise anastomotic suture technique, and careful

Table 1
Results of sleeve pneumonectomy in 8 selected series

Author,[Ref] Year	Number of Patients	Morbidity (%)	Mortality (%)	5-Year Survival (%)
Dartevelle et al,[28] 1995	55	10.8	7.3	40
Mitchell et al,[22] 2001	35	46	20	38
Porhanov et al,[1] 2002	231	35.4	16	19
Regnard et al,[29] 2005	60	54	8.5	26
Raviaro et al,[25] 2006	53	11.3	7.5	33.4
de Perrot,[13] 2006	119	47	7.6	44
Macchiarini et al,[27] 2006	34	16	2	51
Rea et al,[10] 2008	49	28.6	6.1	27.5

handling of tissues are key factors in preventing anastomotic problems.[2]

The role of induction therapy on morbidity and mortality is controversial. de Perrot and colleagues[13] reported an increase in mortality after SP from 6.7% to 13%. On the other hand, Macchiarini and colleagues[27] reported 2% mortality after SP following preoperative chemoradiation.

The reported mortality rates following SP ranges from 2% to 20 % (**Table 1**). In the series reported after 2005, the mortality rate ranges from 2% to 8.5%.[1,10,13,22,25,27–29]

In the authors' center between 2001 and 2010, 12 right and 2 left SPs were performed. Eleven patients were men, with a median age of 62 years (range 41–86 years). Five patients received preoperative chemotherapy and radiotherapy; 3 cases received only preoperative chemotherapy. Partial vena cava superior resection was performed in 3 patients. In 13 patients, the authors wrapped the anastomosis: intercostal flap (n = 6), vena azygos (n = 3), and pericardial fat (n = 4). There was no 30-day mortality. The overall 1-year and 5-year survival rates were 71% and 50%, respectively.

REFERENCES

1. Porhanov VA, Poliakov IS, Selvaschuk AP, et al. Indications and results of sleeve carinal resection. Eur J Cardiothorac Surg 2002;22:685–94.
2. Deslauriers J, Gregoire J, Jacques LF, et al. Sleeve pneumonectomy. Thorac Surg Clin 2004;14:183–90.
3. Abbott OA. Experiences with the surgical of human carina, tracheal wall, and contralateral bronchial wall in cases of right total pneumonectomy. J Thorac Surg 1950;19:906–22.
4. Chamberlain JM, Mc Neill TM, Parnassa P, et al. Bronchogenic carcinoma. an aggressive surgical attitude. J Thorac Surg 1959;38:748.
5. Mathey J, Binet JP, Galey JJ, et al. Tracheal and tracheobronchial resections. Technique and results in 20 cases. J Thorac Cardiovasc Surg 1966;51:1–13.
6. Barclay RS, McSwan N, Welsh TM. Tracheal resection without use of grafts. Thorax 1957;12:177–80.
7. Grillo HC. Carinal reconstruction. Ann Thorac Surg 1982;34:356–73.
8. Mitchell JD. Carinal resection and reconstruction. Chest Surg Clin N Am 2003;13(2):315–29.
9. Lanuti M, Mathisen DJ. Carinal resection. Thorac Surg Clin 2004;14(2):199–209.
10. Rea F, Marulli G, Schiavon M, et al. Tracheal sleeve pneumonectomy for non-small cell lung cancer (NSCLC): Short and long-term results in a single institution. Lung Cancer 2008;61:202–8.
11. Brunelli A, Charloux A, Bolliger CT, et al, European Respiratory Society, European Society of Thoracic Surgeons Joint Task Force on Fitness For Radical Therapy. The European Respiratory Society and European Society of Thoracic Surgeons clinical guidelines for evaluating fitness for radical treatment (surgery and chemoradiotherapy) in patients with lung cancer. Eur J Cardiothorac Surg 2009;36(1):181–4.
12. Dartevelle P, Macchiarini P. Sleeve pneumonectomy. Chest Surg Clin N Am 1999;9(2):407–17.
13. de Perrot M, Fadel E, Mercier O, et al. Long-term results after carinal resection for carcinoma: does the benefit warrant the risk? J Thorac Cardiovasc Surg 2006;131:81–9.
14. Keeyapaj W, Alfirevic A. Carinal resection using an airway exchange catheter-assisted venovenous ECMO technique. Can J Anaesth 2012;59:1075–6.
15. Lei J, Su K, Li XF, et al. Ecmo-assisted carinal resection and reconstruction after left pneumonectomy. J Cardiothorac Surg 2010;5:89–91.
16. Roviaro G, Varoli F, Romanelli A, et al. Complications of tracheal sleeve pneumonectomy: personal experience and overview of the literature. J Thorac Cardiovasc Surg 2001;121(2):234–40.
17. Grillo HC. Carcinoma of the lung: what can be done if the carina is involved? Am J Surg 1982;143(6): 694–5.
18. Abbey Smith R, Nigam BK. Resection of proximal left main bronchus carcinoma. Thorax 1979;34: 616–20.
19. Pearson FG, Todd TR, Cooper JD. Experience with primary neoplasms of the trachea and carina. J Thorac Cardiovasc Surg 1984;88(4):511–8.
20. Mitchell JD, Mathisen DJ, Wright CD, et al. Clinical experience with carinal resection. J Thorac Cardiovasc Surg 1999;117(1):39–52.
21. Bonde P, Papachristos I, McCraith A, et al. Sputum retention after lung operation: prospective, randomized trial shows superiority of prophylactic minitracheostomy in high-risk patients. Ann Thorac Surg 2002;74(1):196–202.
22. Mitchell JD, Mathisen DJ, Wright CD, et al. Resection for bronchogenic carcinoma involving the carina: long-term results and effect of nodal status on outcome. J Thorac Cardiovasc Surg 2001;121(3): 465–71.
23. Deslauriers J, Aucoin A, Grégoire J. Postpneumonectomy pulmonary edema. Chest Surg Clin N Am 1998;8:611–31.
24. Licker M, de Perrot M, Spiliopoulos A, et al. Risk factors for acute lung injury after thoracic surgery for lung cancer. Anesth Analg 2003;97(6):1558–65.
25. Roviaro G, Vergani C, Maciocco M, et al. Tracheal sleeve pneumonectomy: long-term outcome. Lung Cancer 2006;52(1):105–10.
26. Jensik RJ, Faber LP, Kittle CF, et al. Survival in patients undergoing tracheal sleeve pneumonectomy for bronchogenic carcinoma. J Thorac Cardiovasc Surg 1982;84(4):489–96.

27. Macchiarini P, Altmayer M, Go T, et al, Hannover Interdisciplinary Intrathoracic Tumor Task Force Group. Technical innovations of carinal resection for nonsmall-cell lung cancer. Ann Thorac Surg 2006;82(6):1989–97.
28. Dartevelle PG, Macchiarini P, Chapelier AR. 1986: tracheal sleeve pneumonectomy for bronchogenic carcinoma: report of 55 cases. Updated in 1995. Ann Thorac Surg 1995;60(6):1854–5.
29. Regnard JF, Perrotin C, Giovannetti R, et al. Resection for tumors with carinal involvement: technical aspects, results, and prognostic factors. Ann Thorac Surg 2005;80(5):1841–6.

Extended Tracheal Resections

Erich Hecker*, Jan Volmerig

KEYWORDS

• Tracheal resection • Tracheal reconstruction • Extended tracheal resection • Tracheal release

KEY POINTS

- Extended tracheal resection is not only an expression of resected length, but rather a combination of patient parameters (eg, gender, size, habitus, comorbidities), the type of approach (cervical vs sternotomy vs cervical plus [split-]sternotomy, thoracotomy), underlying disease, combination of release maneuvers, and the actual length of necessary tracheal resection.
- The maximum possible length of a tracheal resection can be achieved by using laryngeal release, mobilization of the pretracheal plane, bilateral hilar, and complete pericardial incision.
- Depending on the intraoperative findings, all maneuvers can be performed stepwise so as to achieve a tension-free anastomosis.
- The feasibility of particular steps as minimally invasive, video-assisted measures is yet to be established.
- Although primary short-segment resections (ie, ≤2 cm) generally have good outcomes, the rate of complications in longer resections increases significantly, even in very experienced hands and with release maneuvers.
- Referral to a major center for reoperation after a failed initial attempt is fraught with a high rate of complications and the judgment of an experienced surgeon, both preoperatively and intraoperatively, considering the quality and tension of the tissues is likely to be tremendously important.
- Centers with less volume are urged to consider these facts carefully before undertaking the sporadic case of a potentially longer resection.

EXTENDED TRACHEAL RESECTIONS

The history of tracheal surgery, beginning with the reports of Aretaeus and Galen on tracheostomy in the second and third centuries, is long and slow paced; it was not until the 1950s and following decades that development finally started to accelerate.[1–4]

The reasons for the delayed development were varied. On the one hand, there are a variety of indications for resections:

In non-neoplastic diseases there are post-therapeutic stenosis, postintubation/posttraumatic lesions, idiopathic stenosis, destruction by extratracheal mass, relapsing polychondritis, Wegner granulomatosis, sarcoidosis, amyloidosis, and tracheopathia osteoplastica.

Neoplastic diseases can be distinguished in rare primary tracheal tumors (malignant or benign) and secondary malignant tracheal tumors.

Squamous cell carcinoma and adenoid cystic carcinoma account for two-thirds of primary tracheal tumors, followed by adenocarcinomas, and mucoepidermoid and other mesenchymal carcinomas. Benign tumors are composed of granular cell tumors, fibrous histiocytoma, chondroma, fibroma, hemangioma, and papilloma.

Secondary malignant tumors arise locally from laryngeal structures, thyroid gland, esophagus, lung/bronchi, or as metastatic disease.

The authors declare no competing financial interests.

Department of Thoracic Surgery, Thoraxzentrum Ruhrgebiet, Academic Hospital University Duisburg-Essen, Hordeler Strasse 7-9, Herne 44651, Germany
* Corresponding author.
E-mail address: e.hecker@evk-herne.de

Thorac Surg Clin 24 (2014) 85–95
http://dx.doi.org/10.1016/j.thorsurg.2013.10.005
1547-4127/14/$ – see front matter

thoracic.theclinics.com

The various entities with their varying anatomic locations lead to diverse oncological considerations and tactical strategies, as well as surgical approaches.

Today, in the absence of distant metastasis and if local resectability is provided, primary resection is considered the treatment of choice. If resectability is unclear, operative exploration is to be considered. Primary resection is considered successful in the case of microscopic tumor-bearing resection margins in adenoid cystic carcinomas if local control is supported by postoperative radiation. In addition, in cases of benign neoplasm, endoscopic resection is generally considered the method of choice, for instance laser resection.

The unique features of the trachea with regard to its anatomic location, length, structural rigidity, and blood supply need to be considered by the treating physician.

In 1964, Grillo identified the average length of an adult human trachea to be 11,8 cm, ranging from 10 to 13 cm, and containing 18 to 22 cartilaginous rings, approximately 2 rings per centimeter.[5]

The segmental blood supply of the trachea, first determined by Miura and Grillo in 1966 and later confirmed in detail by Salassa and colleagues, is subject to anatomic descriptions.[6,7]

The first successful bronchial anastomosis was described by Jackson and colleagues in 1949 after accidentally severing a main bronchus.[8] In the same year, based on results from trials in 6 fresh human cadavers, Rob and Bateman estimated the feasible resectability of the trachea to be about 2 cm.[9]

This estimate was strongly advocated by Barclay and colleagues in 1950 and was considered valid for several years.[10]

As a result, there has been considerable effort in developing new materials for tracheal prosthetic replacement, including solid tubes of different materials and rigidity, various mesh-type materials in combination with varying support techniques, as well as wire-reinforced dermal grafts and fascia.

To this day, despite all efforts, no consistent means of tracheal replacement or bridging allowing extended resections has been established.

In 1957, Barclay and colleagues[10] reported of a resection of the carina and proximal right main bronchus, leading to a defect length of 5 cm, which was closed using a new technique of mobilization and bronchial anastomosis with the use of grafts.

In this case, the trachea was fully mobilized within the thorax and the left main bronchus severed from the trachea. After resection of the tumor-bearing area, the right lung was elevated after mobilization by division of the pulmonary ligament. The right main bronchus was anastomosed to the trachea. Reconstruction was completed by insertion of the left main bronchus into the incised intermediate bronchus.

Before this operation, Barclay[10] found that mobilization of the lower trachea, including separation of the left bronchus, facilitated trachea resection to an extent of 6 cm on fresh human cadavers.

In the following decades, research included solutions of primary reconstruction/anastomosis

Table 1
Surgical approaches to tracheal resection

Study	n	Cervical, %	Sternal, %	Thoracic, %
Wright et al,[12] 2004	901	74	20	5
Krajc et al,[13] 2009	164	76	21	—
D'Andrilli et al,[14] 2008	35	100	—	1 minithoracotomy for hilar release
Regnard et al,[15] 1996 multicenter only tumors	208	29	Split 11 Full 36	20
Donahue et al,[16] 1997 Re-resections	75	70	Split 24	3
Rea et al,[31] 2001	65	92	Split 6 Full 2	—
Mutrie et al,[17] 2011	105	93	7	Excluded
Cordos et al,[45] 2008	60	88	Split 5	6
Müller et al,[18–22] 1991	40	55	34	10
Abbasidezfouli et al,[23] 2009	494	—	—	"Few cases"

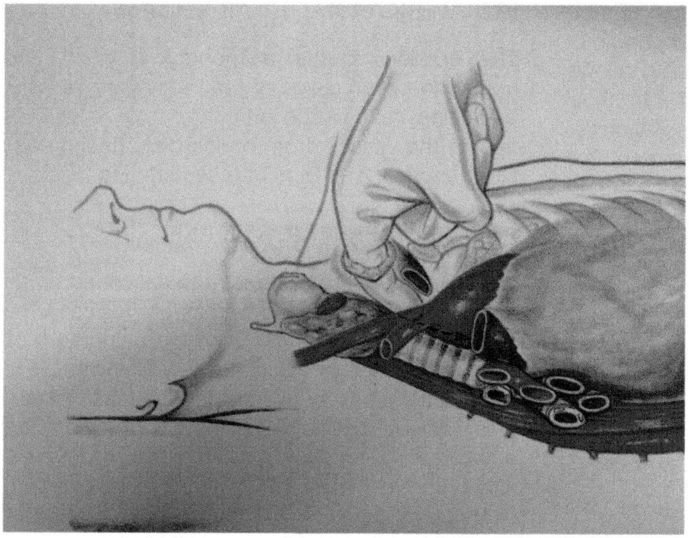

Fig. 1. Digital mobilization of pretracheal plane. (*From* Nier H. Thorax. In: Kremer H, Lierse W, Platzer W, et al, editors. Chirurgische Operationslehre, vol. 2. Germany: Thieme Verlag Stuttgart; 1991. p. 63; with permission.)

after resection, focusing on bearable tension and anatomic mobilization.

Dartevelle recently presented a series of tracheal replacements by forming a tube transplant through cartilage-enforced, vessel, skin, and fascia graft from the forearm and implanting it with revascularization. Although the results are promising, this method is a single-center experience at the moment.[11]

TRACHEAL-RELEASE TECHNIQUES

There is no universally valid definition of the extent of resection that would be considered "extended"; descriptions reach from more than 50% of tracheal length to the use of additional mobilization techniques. A variety of approaches can be used for longer tracheal resections; a split sternotomy is the most common (**Table 1**).

Comments on the interdependency of underlying cause and necessary length of resection, anatomic localization, and chosen surgical approach are found in the discussion section.

MOBILIZATION OF THE PRETRACHEAL PLANE

Digital mobilization of the anterior and anterolateral wall as a basic technique can be performed without devascularization of the trachea. This mobilization can also be performed during video mediastinoscopy as part of oncological staging (**Figs. 1** and **2**). A complete circumferential dissection in a sharp preparation technique is to be limited to about 1 cm next to each side of the intended resection lines to prevent disturbance of blood supply or, depending on the height, injury of the recurrent nerve.

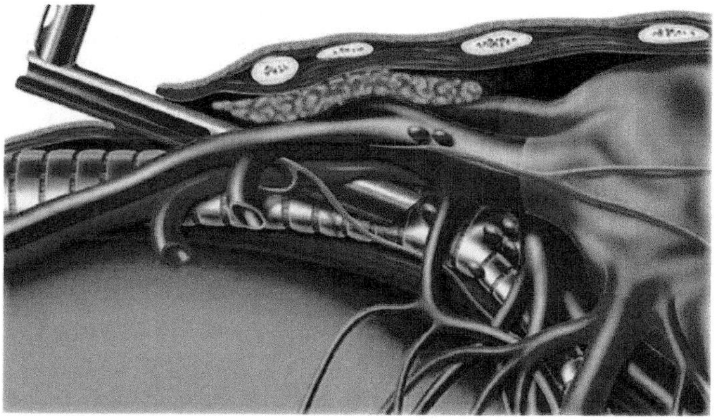

Fig. 2. Mediastinoscopy for mobilization of tracheal plane. (*From* Nier H. Thorax. In: Kremer H, Lierse W, Platzer W, et al, editors. Chirurgische Operationslehre, vol. 2. Germany: Thieme Verlag Stuttgart; 1991. p. 64; with permission.)

Depending on the location of resection, combination with anteflexion of the neck at an angle of 15 to 35° and tension of 1000 to 1200 g allows average resection length of 4.5 cm or 7.2 tracheal rings.[5,24] Many investigators, therefore, favor the securing of neck flexion by chin-to-chest sutures in the initial postoperative course or even a corset in 30° anteflexion.[17,25–33]

SUPRATHYROID LARYNGEAL RELEASE

Described 1969 by Dedo and Fishmann,[34] the suprathyroid laryngeal release method gains a length of approximately 2.0 to 2.5 cm (**Fig. 3**). The thyrohyoid muscles and the thyrohyoid membrane, as well as the ligament, are divided and the tips of the superior cornua are separated under meticulous sparing of superior laryngeal nerves and arteries. The first describing investigators already noted postoperative extensive swallowing problems with high risk of aspiration. The concomitant high incidence of swelling and edema causes surgeons to refrain from this method.

SUPRAHYOID LARYNGEAL RELEASE

In 1974, Montgomery introduced an alternative, less afflicting method of laryngeal release.[35] After dissection of the muscles on the superior surface of the hyoid, the bone itself is divided on each side just anterior to the digastric slings. The drop of larynx measures 2 to 3 cm, allowing additional resection length (**Fig. 4**).

Cervical mobilization techniques are not found to be helpful in influencing the resectable distance in distal/intrathoracic lesions and therefore find their main significance in cervical resections.

INTRAPERICARDIAL HILAR RELEASE

The division of the pulmonary ligament and u-shaped circumcision of the pulmonary vessels, beginning next to the phrenic nerve as well as freeing the vessels from pericardial attachments, allow another 2 + 1 cm of resection (**Fig. 5**).

PERICARDIOPHRENIC RELEASE

The pericardiophrenic release is described as an extended version of the pericardial release. The pericardium is separated from the diaphragm by sharp dissection or electrocautery from ventral to dorsal as well as between the 2 phrenic nerves. This procedure gains another 2 to 3 cm. Postoperative drainage for a few days is considered necessary (**Fig. 6**).

DIVISION OF THE BOTALLI LIGAMENT

Due to the anatomic situation of the left main bronchus and the aortic arch, left-sided hilar release is not as effective as right-sided. The division of the former ductus arteriosus relieves the left main bronchus for mobilization.

REIMPLANTATION OF THE LEFT MAIN BRONCHUS

Using a trans-sternal or preferably a right-sided posterolateral approach, the separation of the left main bronchus using a stapler device liberates the distal trachea and carina, allowing further resection. To avoid length reduction by loss of substance, the bronchus can be just cut off, also allowing an over-the-field jet-ventilation in the separated lung. Reimplantation is performed into the intermediate bronchus at the junction of

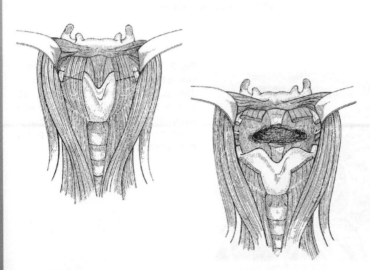

Fig. 3. Suprathyroid laryngeal release. (*Adapted from* Dedo HH, Fishman NH. Laryngeal release and sleeve resection for tracheal stenosis. Ann Otol Rhinol Laryngol 1969;78(2):289; with permission.)

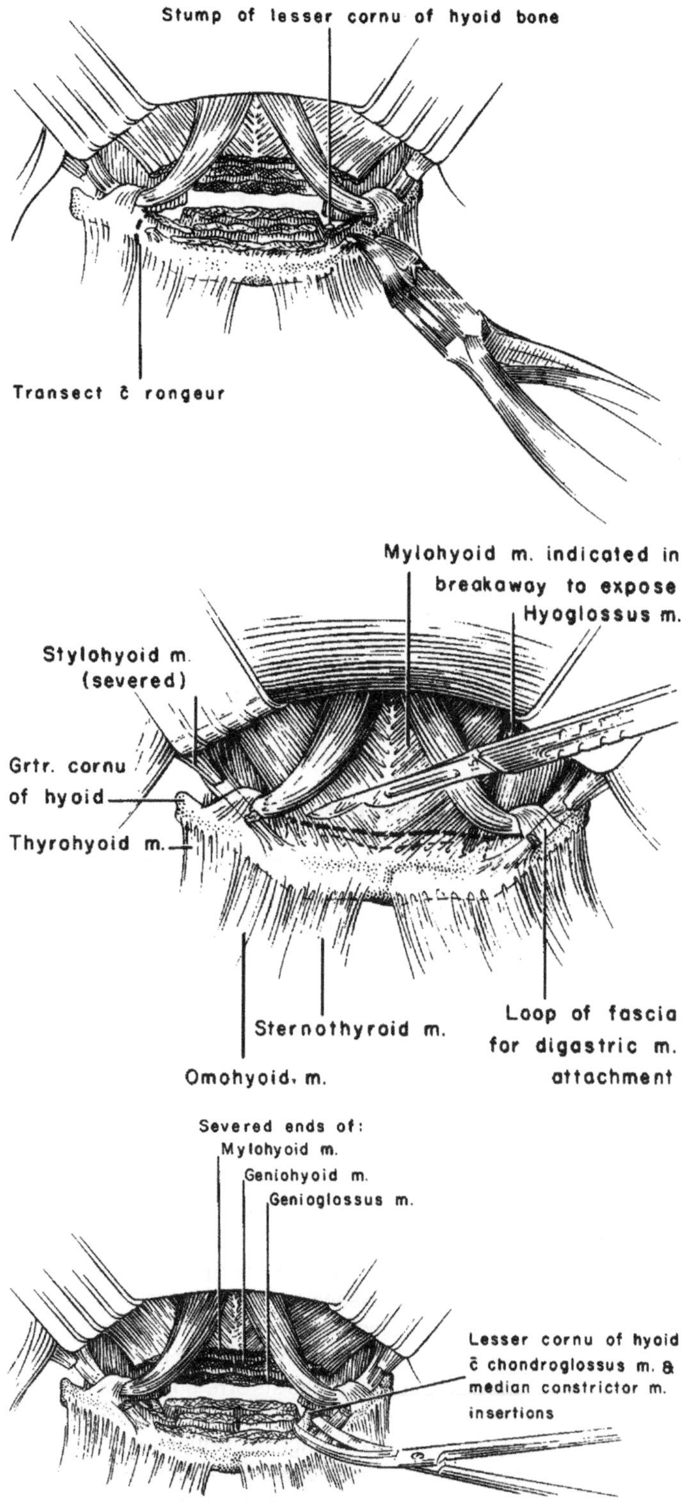

Fig. 4. Suprahyoid laryngeal release. (*Adapted from* Montgomery WW. Suprahyoid release for tracheal anastomosis. Arch Otolaryngol 1974;99(4): 255–56; with permission.)

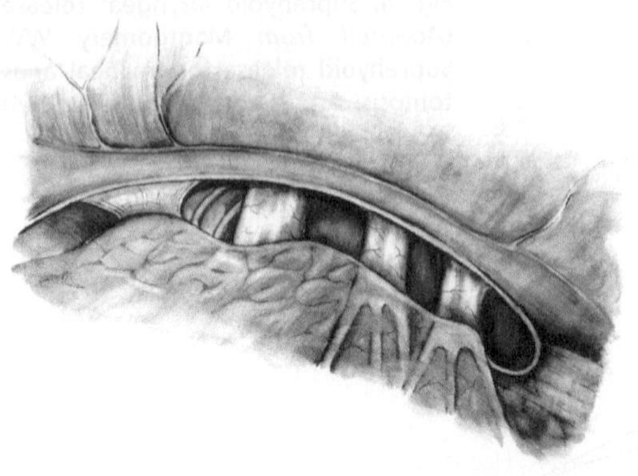

Fig. 5. Hilar mobilization. (*From* Stamatis G. Extensive tracheal resections and reconstruction. Operat Tech Otolaryngol Head Neck Surg 1997;8(3):145; with permission.)

membranous and cartilaginous bronchus after longitudinal incision (**Fig. 7**).

Further techniques of reconstruction are known after carinal resection, which is addressed in the article, "Carinal resection and sleeve pneumonectomy," by Weder and Inci, elsewhere in this issue.

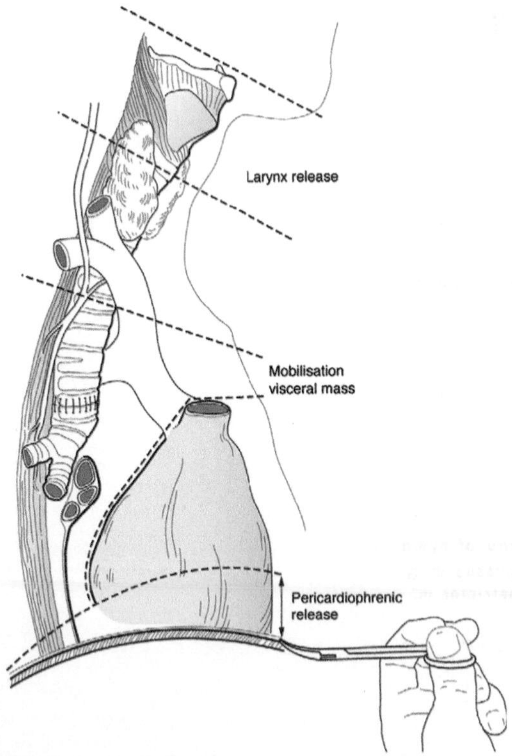

Fig. 6. Pericardiophrenic release. (*From* Macchiarini P, Altmayer M, Go T, et al. Technical Innovations of Carinal Resection for Nonsmall-Cell Lung Cancer: Ann Thorac Surg 2006;82:1992; with permission.)

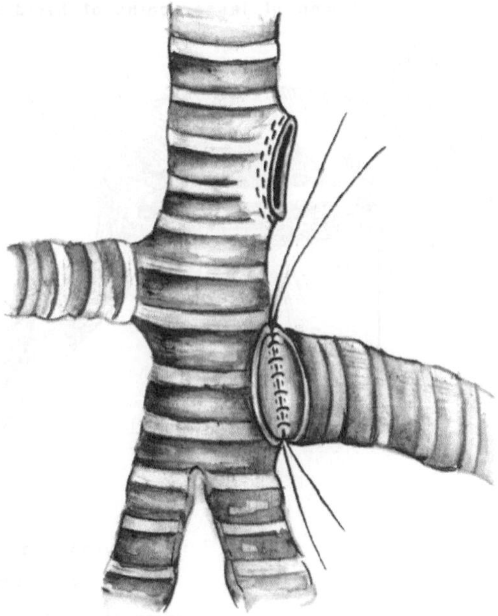

Fig. 7. Reimplantation of the left main bronchus. (*From* Stamatis G. Extensive tracheal resections and reconstruction. Operat Tech Otolaryngol Head Neck Surg 1997;8(3):147; with permission.)

PNEUMOPERITONEUM

This procedure can be considered an anecdote of surgical history, illustrating the imaginative and comprehensive attempts of surgeons. Apart from being a new idea, the negative effects on pulmonary function are bound to exceed the gain in distance. Following the initial description, this method was not pursued in the literature.

RESULTS OF TREATMENT

A variety of complications are reported in tracheal surgery, ranging from early postoperative complications to long-term effects (**Table 2**). A more detailed description is available in the article, "Management of tracheal surgery complications," by Leschber, elsewhere in this issue.

Early anastomotic disruptions are generally uncommon. The treatment depends on the extent of the disruption and consists of re-surgery or stenting.

Other rather early adverse events are neurologic dysphagia and laryngeal dysfunction. The latter is particularly associated with suprathyroid laryngeal release, here caused by extensive swelling and laryngeal edema. Single centers report prophylactic adjuvant therapy for these cases with corticosteroids.[29,36–42]

Laryngeal dysfunction and especially aspiration on deglutition is commonly described as a

Table 2
Results of tracheal resections

Study	n	Excellent and Good Results, %	Resection Length, cm	Separations, %	Release Maneuvers
Wright et al,[12] 2004	901	95	≥4.0 in 31%	9;17 ext. res.	7% laryngeal
Couraud et al,[36] 1995 no tumors	217	96	—	—	—
Krajc et al,[13] 2009	164[a]	94	2.0–6.5	2	—
D'Andrilli et al,[14] 2008	35	86	1.5–6.0 23% ≥ 4.5	3	6% suprahyoid 3% pericardial
Regnard et al,[15] 1996 multicenter only tumors	208	76	3.85 ± 1.4	12	30% laryngeal
Donahue et al,[16] 1997 Re-resections	75	79	1.0–5.5 ~3.5	4	25% 5% thyrohyoid 20% suprahyoid
Rea et al,[31] 2001	65	95	≤4.0	6	1.5% suprahyoid
Mutrie et al,[17] 2011	105	93	1.5–6.0	1	Excl. thoracotomy
Cordos et al,[45] 2008	60	95	1.5–4.0	—	Standard mobilization only
Weidenbecher et al,[29] 2007	101	93	2.0–6.0 4% ≥ 5.0	5	Infrahyoid release if stenosis ≥3 cm
Müller et al,[18] 1991	40	85	1.5–6.5 23% ≥ 4.0	—	—
Abbasidezfouli et al,[23] 2009	494	90 11 Re-stenosis	~3.78 ~4.3	6 infection	"Few cases" suprahyoid + hilar

[a] Only 57% had follow-up information.

temporary or persistent problem after laryngeal release. Most investigators do not differentiate between suprahyoid and suprathyroid release maneuvers or quantify the incidence. In this context, the report of Weidenbecher and colleagues attracts attention.[29] Being an ear, nose, and throat physician, Weidenbecher performed an infrahyoidal release with every resection exceeding a length of 3 cm; he reported a high (not numbered) amount of cases and explicitly mentioned the absence of any long-term disorders. This presentation may be considered a motivation to use this technique when needed.

Vocal cord paralysis is rarely mentioned explicitly, but, if bilateral, can lead to permanent tracheostomy.[17,31]

Pneumonia and respiratory failure and in rare cases cardiac failure are associated with reports of deaths.[12,17,43,44]

Complicating, or even lethal, erosions of the brachiocephalic artery are more often encountered in tracheostomy reports, but also in tracheal resection surgery.[12,45]

Tracheo-esophageal fistula is a possible complication of tracheal resection but it can also be the primary indication for this procedure. Possible mechanisms for the formation are injury to the esophagus that is missed, leading to local infection or anastomotic separation leading to infection and erosion into the esophagus.

The most common problem after tracheal resection is recurrent stenosis, demanding the full spectrum of therapeutic options: reoperation, stenting, dilation, and temporary or permanent tracheostomy/t-tube stenting.[16,23,46–51]

Grillo (1994) set up a classification for judging results in reconstructing tracheal procedures[52]:

Excellent results stand out by anatomically or functionally normal airways. There is no bronchoscopic or radiologic evidence of airway narrowing and the patient suffers no limitations whatsoever.

Narrowing of the airway detectable by bronchoscopy or radiographically without functional impairment of the patient is considered *good*.

Satisfactory results permit patients all regular daily activities but limiting them in major physical efforts.

All other outcomes, including the death of the patient, are considered and summarized as *failures*.

Literature specifically on postoperative results of extended tracheal surgery is scarce. Most existing publications either focus on the results of tracheal resection in general or on the varying underlying causes for the intervention, such a as tumor or stenosis.

In the context of a national multicenter retrospective study on resected primary tracheal tumors, Regnard and colleagues,[15] on behalf of the French Society of Thoracic and Cardiovascular Surgery, reported 165 resections with primary anastomosis in 1995.[53,54] Length of resection (in resection lengths 38.5 ± 14.0 mm), as well as the need for laryngeal release, was found to be significantly associated with postoperative complications, but not further allocated.

In 1997, Stamatis published his experience with 33 patients with extended tracheal resection of more than half of the trachea for various pathologies, using various mobilization techniques.[55] Although the results show a very positive overall outcome (66%, 21/32 excellent in the Grillo classification), the variables length, localization, and method of mobilization are neither documented nor analyzed.

The most comprehensive publication was published by Wright and colleagues,[12] including a total of 901 patients and a multivariable analysis. In this, resection lengths of 4 cm or longer could be identified as an independent risk factor, dramatically increasing the failure rate (**Fig. 8**). Anastomotic failure in primary resection of 4 cm or longer was found to be even more frequent than complication rates of secondary operations after failures of primary resection of less than 2.5-cm length.[12]

Unfortunately, the investigators did not correlate outcome with surgical technique or mobilization technique. Laryngeal releases were explicitly excluded from an individual consideration as a risk factor, with the striking argument that clinical need for release because of resection length otherwise would lead to excessive tension if not performed, thus having 2 variables in contest. Among resections that required a laryngeal release, the rate of separation (requiring stent, t-tube, or reoperation) was 27% despite the release, even in these experienced hands. Other methods of mobilization were not addressed specifically.

In an institutional report, Krajc and colleagues[13] outline 164 cases of resection due to benign stenosis or lesions. Depending on localization and underlying etiology, subglottic and upper third tracheal lesion were resected by transcervical approach, middle third tracheal region by sternotomy, and lower third by thoracotomy. Resection lengths were up to 6.5 cm in all locations, information on mobilization techniques was not provided.[13]

As an example for a more recent publication, Mutrie and colleagues[17] summed up 105 patients with 108 resections for various pathologies. They report of resection lengths of up to 6 cm, focusing

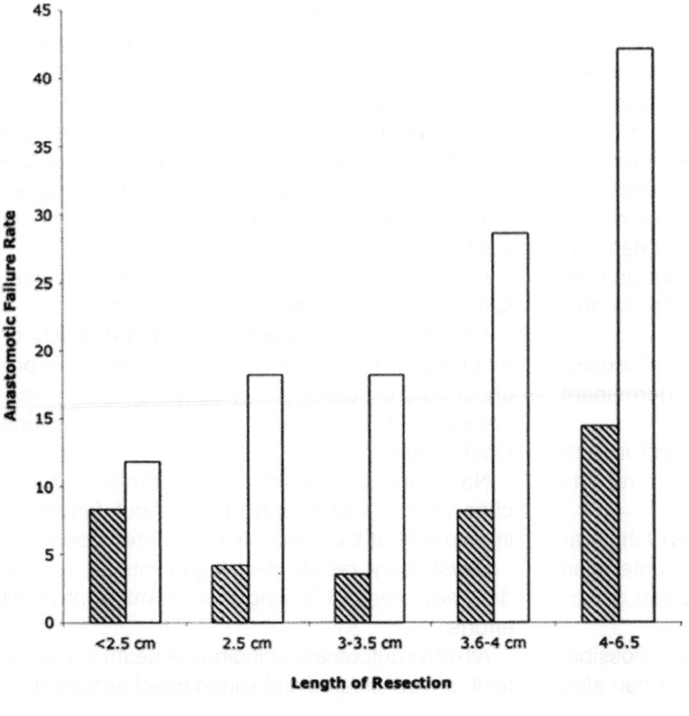

Fig. 8. Anastomotic complication rate as function of length of tracheal resection in patients undergoing first resection (n = 800, *diagonally striped bars*) and reoperation (n = 101, *solid bars*). Lengths are presented as quintiles. (*From* Wright CD, Grillo HC, Wain JC, et al. Anastomotic complications after tracheal resection: prognostic factors and management. J Thorac Cardiovasc Surg 2004;128(5):731–9; with permission.)

on tracheal resections and excluding potentially necessary thoracotomy but including an upper partial sternotomy. Of the listed mobilization techniques, dissection of the pretracheal plane down to the carina and a suprahyoid laryngeal release were applied. In this study, resection length had no prognostic impact and mobilization techniques were not considered separately.[17]

Tracheal resections are influenced by patient age, gender, habitus, prior surgery, comorbidity, and the underlying disease, but also by experience of the surgeon and the anesthesiologist in airway management and oxygenation techniques.

This variety affords interdisciplinary, personalized planning, as well as a broad spectrum of applicable surgical techniques on behalf of the surgeon considering the chosen approach, targeted surgical result, and surgical alternatives in the course of the procedure.

Most necessary resections affect the cervical trachea and can be performed as primary resection with anastomosis, without the aid of mobilization techniques.

Trachea resectability is influenced not only by the localization to be resected as well as the previously mentioned items, but also possible tracheal calcification or fibrosis of the "healthy" intercartilaginous structures leading to shortening. For this, resection length may be a poor benchmark for comparison.

On the other hand, resection length of 4 cm or longer has been identified as an individual risk factor with an odds ratio of 2.01 and increasing the rate of anastomosis separation from 9% to 17%.[12] Correspondent to this fact and the reviewed data, the investigators suggest this length to be literally considered a "cutoff margin" for the definition of an extended tracheal resection.

Surgeons performing tracheal surgery should be familiar with technical possibilities and limitations. Careful preoperative planning is essential for successful management of unsuspected intraoperative findings or deviations from the planned strategy.

Tension of the anastomosis is undoubtedly a major risk factor for an unfavorable postoperative course. The correct judgment of the necessary extent of the release maneuvers is one of the main technical skills a surgeon should hold.

Dissection of the pretracheal plane is the most common form of release. Laryngeal release is focused on suprahyoid mobilization, but is still affiliated with functional problems.

Thoracic mobilization is generally not considered to be favorable for cervical resection, but with resection of greater lengths that involve more of the thoracic trachea, they may sometimes be helpful.

As Wright and colleagues[12] clearly emphasized in their discussion, there is an area of conflict in the interpretation of the necessity of mobilization by the surgeon due to the resection length/tension of the anastomosis and the outcome, anticipating an excessive failure rate if mobilization was not performed.

On the other hand, surgeons may limit themselves in the options of mobilization, dreading a sternal or thoracic approach. In the opinion of the authors, the enormous advances in video-assisted thoracoscopic techniques during the past decades have opened further possibilities for minimally invasive thoracic mobilization (eg, combination of video-assisted thoracoscopic surgery and mediastinoscopic approach), which have yet to be explored and put into practice. It may be of great interest and subject to further examinations, to what extent a limited thoracoscopic mobilization of the hilum and pulmonary ligament and/or pericardium can further reduce anastomosis tension.

SUMMARY

Extended tracheal resection is not only an expression of resected length. It is rather a combination of patient parameters (eg, gender, size, habitus, comorbidities), the type of approach (cervical vs sternotomy vs cervical plus [split-]sternotomy, thoracotomy), underlying disease, combination of release maneuvers, and the actual length of necessary tracheal resection.

A length of less than 4 cm can be considered an approximated "cutoff margin" for "standard" tracheal resections. Beyond this, complications are more likely and release maneuvers often necessary to achieve tension-limited anastomosis. The maximum possible length of a tracheal resection can be achieved by using laryngeal release, mobilization of the pretracheal plane, and bilateral hilar, as well as complete pericardial incision.

In the authors' opinion, a maximum of 7 cm of tissue deficiency in addition to and dependency of the patient-specific tracheal elasticity is bridgeable. All surgical procedures are technically feasible in the supine position. Depending on the intraoperative findings, all maneuvers can be performed stepwise so as to achieve a tension-free anastomosis. The feasibility of particular steps as a minimally invasive, video-assisted measure is yet to be established.

Extended tracheal resection should be performed only in centers that feel comfortable in performing all possibly necessary (open and minimally invasive [video-assisted]) procedures for mobilization safely. Although primary short-segment resections (ie, ≤2 cm) generally have good outcomes, the rate of complications in longer resections increases significantly, even in very experienced hands and with release maneuvers. The judgment of an experienced surgeon, both preoperatively and intraoperatively, considering the quality and tension of the tissues, is likely to be tremendously important. Furthermore, referral to a major center for reoperation after a failed initial attempt is fraught with a high rate of complications. Centers with less volume are urged to consider these facts carefully before undertaking the sporadic case of a potentially longer resection.

REFERENCES

1. Bagheri R, Majidi M, Khadivi E, et al. Outcome of surgical treatment for proximal long segment post intubation tracheal stenosis. J Cardiothorac Surg 2013;8:35.
2. Linder A, Busemann A, Menges P. 100 years resection of the complete trachea. Zentralbl Chir 2013; 138(1):107–10 [in German].
3. Muniappan A, Wain JC, Wright CD, et al. Surgical treatment of nonmalignant tracheoesophageal fistula: a thirty-five year experience. Ann Thorac Surg 2013;95(4):1141–6.
4. Grillo HC. Development of tracheal surgery: a historical review. Part 1: techniques of tracheal surgery. Ann Thorac Surg 2003;75:610–9.
5. Grillo HC, Dignan EF, Miura T. Extensive resection and reconstruction of mediastinal trachea without prosthesis or graft: an anatomical study in man. J Thorac Cardiovasc Surg 1964;48:741–9.
6. Salassa JR, Pearson BW, Payne WS. Gross and microscopical blood supply of the trachea. Ann Thorac Surg 1977;24:100–7.
7. Miura T, Grillo HC. The contribution of the inferior thyroid artery to the blood supply of the human trachea. Surg Gynecol Obstet 1966;123:99.
8. Jackson TL, Lefkin P, et al. An experimental study in bronchial anastomosis. J Thorac Surg 1949;18(5): 630–42.
9. Rob CG, Bateman GH. Reconstruction of the trachea and cervical esophagus. Br J Surg 1949;37: 202–5.
10. Barclay RS, McSwan N, Welsh TM. Tracheal reconstruction without the use of grafts. Thorax 1957;12: 177–80.
11. Fabre D, Kolb F, Fadel E, et al. Successful tracheal replacement in humans using autologous tissues: an 8-year experience. Ann Thorac Surg 2013; 96(4):1146–55.
12. Wright CD, Grillo HC, Wain JC, et al. Anastomotic complications after tracheal resection: prognostic factors and management. J Thorac Cardiovasc Surg 2004;128(5):731–9.
13. Krajc T, Janik M, Benej R, et al. Urgent segmental resection as the primary strategy in management of benign tracheal stenosis. A single center experience in 164 consecutive cases. Interact Cardiovasc Thorac Surg 2009;9:983–9.
14. D'Andrilli A, Ciccone AM, Venuta F, et al. Long-term results of laryngotracheal resection for benign stenosis. Eur J Cardiothorac Surg 2008;33(3):440–3.
15. Regnard JF, Fourquier P, Levasseur P. Results and prognostic factors in resections of primary tracheal tumors: a multicenter retrospective study. The French Society of Cardiovascular Surgery. J Thorac Cardiovasc Surg 1996;111(4):808–13.
16. Donahue DM, Grillo HC, Wain JC, et al. Reoperative tracheal resection and reconstruction for unsuccessful repair of postintubation stenosis. J Thorac Cardiovasc Surg 1997;114(6):934–8 [discussion: 938–9].
17. Mutrie CJ, Eldaif SM, Rutledge CW, et al. Cervical tracheal resection: new lessons learned. Ann Thorac Surg 2011;91(4):1101–6 [discussion: 1106].
18. Müller MR, Klepetko W, Rogy M, et al. Results of transverse tracheal resection in post-intubation tracheal stenoses. Chirurg 1991;62(7):547–51 [in German].
19. París F, Borro JM, Tarrazona V, et al. Management of non-tumoral tracheal stenosis in 112 patients. Eur J Cardiothorac Surg 1990;4(5):265–8 [discussion: 268–9].
20. Grillo HC, Mathisen DJ. Primary tracheal tumors: treatment and results. Ann Thorac Surg 1990;49(1): 69–77.
21. von Glass W, Weidenbecher M. Early and long-term results following tracheal segment resection. HNO 1989;37(6):259–63 [in German].
22. Heberer G, Schildberg FW, Valesky A, et al. Trachea reconstruction in inflammatory stenosis and tumors. Chirurg 1980;51(5):283–90 [in German].
23. Abbasidezfouli A, Akbarian E, Shadmehr BM, et al. The etiological factors of recurrence after tracheal resection and reconstruction in post-intubation stenosis. Interact Cardiovasc Thorac Surg 2009;9: 446–9.
24. Mulliken JB, Grillo HC. The limits of tracheal resection with primary anastomosis. J Thorac Cardiovasc Surg 1968;55:418–21.
25. Hoerbelt R, Padberg W. Primary tracheal tumors of the neck and mediastinum resection and reconstruction procedures. Chirurg 2011;82(2):125–33 [in German].
26. D'Andrilli A, Rendina EA, Venuta F. Tracheal surgery. Monaldi Arch Chest Dis 2010;73(3):105–15.
27. Macchiarini P, Rovira I, Ferrarello S. Awake upper airway surgery. Ann Thorac Surg 2010;89(2): 387–90 [discussion: 390–1].

28. Wain JC Jr. Postintubation tracheal stenosis. Semin Thorac Cardiovasc Surg 2009;21(3):284–9.
29. Weidenbecher M Jr, Weidenbecher M, Iro H. Segmental tracheal resection for the treatment of tracheal stenoses. HNO 2007;55(1):21–8.
30. Gaissert HA, Grillo HC, Shadmehr MB, et al. Long-term survival after resection of primary adenoid cystic and squamous cell carcinoma of the trachea and carina. Ann Thorac Surg 2004;78(6):1889–96 [discussion: 1896–7].
31. Rea F, Callegaro D, Loy M, et al. Benign tracheal and laryngotracheal stenosis: surgical treatment and results. Eur J Cardiothorac Surg 2002;22(3):352–6.
32. Acosta AC, Albanese CT, Farmer DL, et al. Tracheal stenosis: the long and the short of it. J Pediatr Surg 2000;35(11):1612–6.
33. Jalal A, Jeyasingham K. Bronchoplasty for malignant and benign conditions: a retrospective study of 44 cases. Eur J Cardiothorac Surg 2000;17(4):370–6.
34. Dedo HH, Fishman NH. Laryngeal release and sleeve resection for tracheal stenosis. Ann Otol Rhinol Laryngol 1969;78(2):285–96.
35. Montgomery WW. Suprahyoid release for tracheal anastomosis. Arch Otolaryngol 1974;99(4):255–60.
36. Couraud L, Jougon JB, Velly JF. Surgical treatment of nontumoral stenoses of the upper airway. Ann Thorac Surg 1995;60(2):250–9 [discussion: 259–60].
37. Zwischenberger JB, Sankar AB. Surgery of the thoracic trachea. J Thorac Imaging 1995;10(3):199–205.
38. Mansour KA, Lee RB, Miller JI Jr. Tracheal resections: lessons learned. Ann Thorac Surg 1994;57(5):1120–4 [discussion: 1124–5].
39. Macchiarini P, Chapelier A, Lenot B, et al. Laryngotracheal resection and reconstruction for postintubation subglottic stenosis. Lessons learned. Eur J Cardiothorac Surg 1993;7(6):300–5.
40. Maddaus MA, Toth JL, Gullane PJ, et al. Subglottic tracheal resection and synchronous laryngeal reconstruction. J Thorac Cardiovasc Surg 1992;104(5):1443–50.
41. Bisson A, Bonnette P, el Kadi NB, et al. Tracheal sleeve resection for iatrogenic stenoses (subglottic laryngeal and tracheal). J Thorac Cardiovasc Surg 1992;104(4):882–7.
42. Grillo HC, Mathisen DJ, Wain JC. Laryngotracheal resection and reconstruction for subglottic stenosis. Ann Thorac Surg 1992;53(1):54–63.
43. Cuisnier O, Righini Ch, Pison Ch, et al. Surgical and/or endoscopic treatment of acquired tracheal stenosis in adult patients. Ann Otolaryngol Chir Cervicofac 2004;121(1):3–13.
44. Donahue DM. Reoperative tracheal surgery. Chest Surg Clin N Am 2003;13(2):375–83.
45. Cordos I, Bolca C, Paleru C, et al. Sixty tracheal resections—single center experience. Interact Cardiovasc Thorac Surg 2009;8(1):62–5 [discussion: 65].
46. Maziak DE, Todd TR, Keshavjee SH, et al. Adenoid cystic carcinoma of the airway: thirty-two-year experience. J Thorac Cardiovasc Surg 1996;112(6):1522–31 [discussion: 1531–2].
47. Laccourreye O, Naudo P, Brasnu D, et al. Tracheal resection with end-to-end anastomosis for isolated postintubation cervical trachea stenosis: long-term results. Ann Otol Rhinol Laryngol 1996;105(12):944–8.
48. Mathisen DJ. Complications of tracheal surgery. Chest Surg Clin N Am 1996;6(4):853–64.
49. Grillo HC, Donahue DM. Postintubation tracheal stenosis. Chest Surg Clin N Am 1996;6(4):725–31.
50. Heitmiller RF. Tracheal release maneuvers. Chest Surg Clin N Am 1996;6(4):675–82.
51. Pearson FG, Gullane P. Subglottic resection with primary tracheal anastomosis: including synchronous laryngotracheal reconstructions. Semin Thorac Cardiovasc Surg 1996;8(4):381–91.
52. Grillo HC. Management of non-neoplastic diseases of the trachea. In: Schields TW, editors. General thoracic surgery. Baltimore (MD): Williams.
53. Regnard JF, Fourquier P, Levasseur P. Resections of primary tracheal tumors: a multicenter retrospective study. The French Society of Cardiovascular Surgery. J Thorac Cardiovasc Surg 1996;111(4):808–13 [discussion: 813–4].
54. Sharpe DA, Moghissi K. Tracheal resection and reconstruction: a review of 82 patients. Eur J Cardiothorac Surg 1996;10(12):1040–5 [discussion: 1045–6].
55. Stamatis G. Extensive tracheal resections and reconstruction. Operat Tech Otolaryngol Head Neck Surg 1997;8:142–8.

Airway Transplantation

Philipp Jungebluth, Paolo Macchiarini*

KEYWORDS

• Trachea replacement • Tissue engineering • Allogenic transplantation
• Immunosuppressive medication • Rejection

KEY POINTS

- Replacing long segments or the entire trachea in humans.
- Allotransplantation.
- Surgical challenges.
- Organ rejection.
- Tissue engineering.

A variety of benign or malignant disorders affecting the trachea can theoretically be treated by simple resection and subsequent end-to-end anastomosis of the remaining trachea.[1] This primary reconstruction is, so far, the only curative treatment in patients with tracheal diseases but, unfortunately, it is feasible only when the affected tracheal length does not exceed 6 cm in adults and about 30% of the entire length in children. Besides this technical restriction, local anatomy, previous treatments, and type of pathologic condition can further restrict the already few therapeutic options.

Longer segments cannot be treated surgically because it is impossible to perform safely a direct reconstruction of the airway that, under these circumstances, would ultimately fail because of the excessive tension at the anastomotic site. Benign diseases have been approached with various endoluminal solutions.[1,2] Because most of primary tracheal malignancies are diagnosed in an advanced local stage, only palliative options remain available, such as stenting, tumor debulking or radiotherapy.[1,3] Consequently, tracheal transplantation could be a valid alternative for many patients (**Table 1**). To this end, different replacement strategies have been investigated in experimental settings and some of them translated to the clinic. However, so far, none of them has turned into a routine clinical procedure. The requirements of an ideal tracheal substitute are multifaceted but crucial for a successful clinical application (**Table 2**).

TYPES OF TRANSPLANTATIONS

In 1963, Fonkalsrud and Sumida,[4] and, in 1971, Fonkalsrud and colleagues,[5] reported two initial clinical cases of tracheal replacement using the patients' own esophagus in congenital agenesis and long-segment stenosis. Initially, the patients recovered remarkably but then died within the first 6 weeks postoperatively. Both neotrachea required permanent stenting and did not provide normal

The authors declare no competing financial interests.
This work was supported by European Project FP7-NMP- 2011-SMALL-5, BIOtrachea; Bio- materials for Tracheal Replacement in Age-related Cancer via a Humanly Engineered Airway (No. 280584e2); ALF medicine (Stockholm County Council), Transplantation of Bioengineered Trachea in Humans (No. LS1101e0042); The Swedish Heart-Lung Foundation, Trachea Tissue Engineering; Doctor Dorka Stiftung (Hannover, Germany), bioengineering of tracheal tissue; and a megagrant of the Russian Ministry of Education and Science (agreement No. 11.G34.31.0065).
Division of Ear, Nose, and Throat (CLINTEC), Advanced Center for Translational Regenerative Medicine (ACTREM), Karolinska Institutet, Alfred Nobel Allé 8, Huddinge/Stockholm 14186, Sweden
* Corresponding author.
E-mail address: paolo.macchiarini@ki.se

Thorac Surg Clin 24 (2014) 97–106
http://dx.doi.org/10.1016/j.thorsurg.2013.09.005
1547-4127/14/$ – see front matter

Table 1
Indications for potential tracheal transplantation and eligibility criteria

Indications	Benign Diseases	Malignant Diseases
—	• Trauma • Benign stenosis • Relapsing polychondritis • Osteochondroplastica • Amyloidosis • Tuberculosis	• Unresectable tumors • Postlaryngectomy recurrences or diseases
	Eligibility Criteria	
	• Extended (>60% total length) benign & malignant diseases • Already maximally pretreated • Age between 10 and 75 y • No absolute surgical contraindications • No regional and/or micrometastasis (bone-marrow biopsy proven) • Normal psychological or psychiatric habitus • Independent review board, ethics and national transplant clearance • Written informed consent	

function. No similar transplants have been made since. Instead, a variety of approaches have been attempted clinically that use either allotransplantation or tissue engineering (TE) approaches.

TRACHEAL ALLOTRANSPLANTATION

Fresh Cadaveric Trachea

In 1979, Rose and colleagues[6] described the first case of allogenic tracheal replacement using a fresh cadaveric tracheal graft in a 21-year-old male patient with extensive benign tracheal stenosis. In a two-stage procedure, the graft was initially implanted into the sternocleidomastoid muscle region to provide indirect vascularization and subsequently transferred to the orthotopic site. The patient was discharged 9 weeks after the transplantation without immunosuppressive medication and no signs for organ rejection or health status impairment. At that time, it was assumed that the tracheal immunogenicity was not relevant and graft failure was only provoked by graft ischemia and infection.[6] In contrast, Levashov and colleagues[7] transplanted on a donated trachea but with different findings. They used the omentopexy to obtain indirect blood supply of the cadaveric trachea and reported signs of organ rejection at day 10 postoperatively. The investigators affirmed the promising overall outcome 4 months after the transplantation but emphasized the essential need of adequate donor-recipient selection and modern immunosuppressive medication. Similar

Table 2
Requirements of ideal tracheal substitute

Scaffold for Tissue Replacement	Characteristics
General properties	• Nonimmunogenic • Nontoxic • Nontumorigenic • Allows for cell adhesion, migration, proliferation, and differentiation
Tracheal-specific properties	• Airtight and liquid-tight seals • Mechanical properties to react on both lateral and • Longitudinal forces • Support airway patency and respiratory function
Required mechanical properties based on native trachea	± 75° (right/left axial rotation at 0° maximum flexion) ± 75° (right/left axial rotation at 0° flexion) Flexion/extension 70°/60° and 40% of strain limit (flexion-extension bending) 40%:20% for tension/compression (axial/tension/compression) Lateral (right/left) bending: 48° and expected strain limit of 40%

findings were obtained by Delaere and colleagues[8] in a small animal model confirming the necessity of immunosuppressive medication for tracheal transplantation. In another in-depth evaluation of the antigenic profile of the human trachea, Shaari and colleagues[9] discovered the underlying mechanism of the immune competence of human trachea.

Despite the obvious significance of immunogenicity, most research was focused on graft revascularization. Klepetko and colleagues[10] demonstrated that the structural and functional properties of an allogenic graft could be maintained with heterotopic transplantation into the omentum. In a large animal study, Macchiarini and colleagues[11] described a harvesting technique to revascularize the entire trachea that, to be successful, required heavy immunosuppression to control rejection and perfect venous drainage. This experience has been applied by Duque and colleagues,[12] in Columbia, who have reported a series of 20 clinical laryngeal and tracheal transplants. An extension of this technique, a composite laryngotracheal (7 cm) graft transplant, was recently used in a 51-year-old woman already on immunosuppression.[13] Postoperatively, the patient continues to rely on a tracheotomy but has had the return of an oral and nasal airway, vocalization, smell, and taste.

The pros of this method are excellent vascularity and maintenance of functional integrity. The cons include life-long heavy immunosuppression and donor dependence.

In Situ Processed Fresh Cadaveric Trachea

Like Rose and colleagues,[6] Delaere and colleagues[14] investigated the interesting approach of using fresh cadaveric allografts. The harvested trachea was initially transplanted into the subcutaneous tissue of the recipient's forearm to induce neovascularization of the graft. Meanwhile, immunosuppressive medication was initiated and continued for the next 229 days. Within the observation period, the posterior wall of the heterotopic implanted graft became necrotic, and was removed and replaced by buccal mucosa of the recipient. After 4 months, the allograft was placed into the orthotopic position and a 4.5 cm defect of the patient's trachea replaced. At the time of orthotopic transplantation, the graft showed cartilage rings composed of viable cartilage tissue and epithelial lining consisting of squamous epithelium and respiratory epithelium.

The pro of this method is the need for immunosuppression is only early, not life-long. The cons are long-lasting and multiple procedures. So far, only short-segment replacement could be resected using standard techniques.

Cryopreserved, Irradiated, or Chemically Preserved Trachea

To avoid immunosuppressive medication, various attempts to reduce graft immunogenicity, such as cryopreservation,[15] irradiation, or detergent enzymatic treatment were investigated. Unfortunately, it was soon evident that the mechanical and structural macroscopic properties and cell adhesion and behavior would be damaged.[15–18] The long processing time was also a concern, especially for patients with malignancies. Regarding chemically fixated tracheae, Jacobs and colleagues[19] reported on 131 patients (100 adults and 31 children) who were treated with such processed grafts.[20] The technique was only applied in patients with benign tracheal disorders, except for one who had adenoid cystic carcinoma, with satisfactory results. However, because it requires an intact posterior tracheal wall, this technique is unfeasible for extended circumferential malignancies. The common denominator of these reconstructive methods is the need of permanent stenting. The pro of these methods is that there is no need for immunosuppressive medication. The cons are that they are donor dependent, have an extended processing time, are partly posterior wall dependent, involve stenting, and are nonvital.

Fresh or Cryopreserved Cadaveric Aorta

Some groups investigated the use of aortic grafts to replace the affected part of the windpipe. Carbognani and colleagues[21] introduced the technique of using a cryopreserved aortic allograft. Their study showed the technical feasibility of the method but also the imperative necessity of always placing a permanent stent into the graft to provide normal function and limit fibroblasts colonization. Wurtz and colleagues[22] reported satisfying clinical results without immunosuppressive medication by using either fresh or cryopreserved aortic homografts.[23] Nevertheless, the lack of cartilage-ring development and, therefore, related loss of structural integrity requires permanent stenting and other mechanical support.[22,24] The pro for these methods is that there is no need for immunosuppressive medication. The cons are donor dependence and permanent intraluminal stenting.

TE

Hermes Grillo,[1] a pioneer of airway surgery, stated that TE could become the most promising therapeutic concept for patients with inoperable tracheal lesions. Experimental studies demonstrated the potential of TE for nearly every solid or tubular organ and each type of tissue. Initial clinical applications for a variety of these, such as heart valves, urine bladder, tubular structures, suggest the technologic feasibility and potential.[25–28] The concept of TE is based on four components: (1) scaffold or matrix, (2) cells, (3) bioreactor, and (4) various bioactive molecules.

The Scaffold

The scaffold is the basic component that provides the structural integrity of the graft. Characteristics must meet both general and organ requirements, including trachea-specific criteria. General requirements are that it is nonimmunogenic, nontoxic, and nontumorigenic, as well as allows for cell adhesion, migration, proliferation, and differentiation. Trachea-specific characteristics include airtight and liquid-tight seals at the start; mechanical properties that will react on both lateral and longitudinal forces, and support airway patency; and adequate respiratory function.

The biologic scaffold

Various biologic scaffolds have been investigated for their potential use but the ideal scaffold source depends on the target tissue. For the trachea in particular, three natural tissues have been tested in detail: the trachea,[29–31] porcine jejunum,[32] and the aorta.[33] The primary goal of TE is to provide a nonimmunogenic scaffold that can be transplanted without any subsequent need of immunosuppressive medication. Because the major histocompatibility complexes I and II are key for adverse immune reaction, it is imperative to remove them from the donor tissue. Decellularization, using various methods such as detergent and enzymatic solutions (ionic, nonionic, resolvent, chelating, alkaline, acidic, zwitterionic) and/or physical methods (perfusion, agitation, static), has demonstrated its efficiency in doing so. During the removal of the genomic DNA, the nanofiber architecture of the extracellular matrix (ECM) remained intact and the bioengineered ECM consisted of several proteins (laminin, elastin, collagen) of significant importance for cell homing, differentiation, migration, and proliferation. Each decellularization strategy has a different impact on the in vivo degradation process of the ECM, which essentially influences tissue remodeling stimulation, angiogenesis (neoformation of vessels), and cell homing.

To date, initial cases of clinical transplantation using biologic scaffolds processed by detergent enzymatic method have been reported with promising early outcome for both a decellularized trachea[27,34] and a porcine jejunum.[32,35] Macchiarini and colleagues performed a series that included nine patients suffering from various disorders and treated with a decellularized and reseeded trachea. Notably, they recognized unpredicted mechanical impairments within 12 months in about 30% of the patients (Macchiarini, personal communication, 2013). The pros of this method are that there is no need for immunosuppressive medication and preservation of the ECM. The cons are donor dependency, processing time, and biomechanical degeneration.

The artificial scaffold

Even though the initial clinical experience with biologic scaffolds seems promising, drawbacks do still exist, even though the biologic scaffolds do yet require a human donation. The decellularization protocol lasts approximately 2 to 3 weeks, which might not be practical for patients with malignant diseases that require an early treatment. In addition, the mechanical properties are a disadvantage, particularly for longer segments that require recurrent stenting because of the clinically observed instable biomechanics. Therefore, other alternatives are more desired.

As discussed previously, the assumption that the trachea is only a tubular structure to transport air from the larynx to the lungs is obsolete; other functions and characteristics have been elucidated. This complexity explains why synthetic grafts failed in serving as tracheal grafts.

> *Only a living substitute, therefore vascularized, can pretend to fulfill the anatomic mechanical and anti-infectious functions of the trachea.*
>
> —*Macchiarini*[36]

Artificial material that is not vascularized and is nonvital incorporates a low level of integrity, indicates a trend for migration and contamination, and is usually rather stiff and nonflexible. The absence of vascularization and immunocompetence must be solved to overcome all drawbacks of synthetic materials and their associated complications.[1]

Why artificial?

Synthetic scaffolds have unlimited availability, can be customized and manufactured to meet the patients needs, are inexpensive and fast to process, and can be sterilized without altering cell biology. Various biodegradable and nondegradable materials have been evaluated, including Marlex mesh (Chevron Phillips Chemical Company LP, TX, USA), polyethylene oxide/polypropylene oxide copolymer (Pluronic F-127, Invitrogen, Ltd,

Paisley, UK), polyester urethane, polyethylene glycol–based hydrogel, polyhydroxy acids, poly-ε-caprolactone, polypropylene mesh, poly (lactic–co-glycolic acid) polymer, gelatin sponge, and alginate gel.[1] To date only few clinical applications have been reported using synthetic based scaffolds.[37–39]

Various matters must be considered to turn synthetic materials into viable tissue. Aside from using cells to reseed the scaffold, pharmaceutical interventions are crucial to support the regeneration of the implanted graft. Moreover, the blood supply can be provided by indirect vascularization via surgical techniques, such as with the omentum major, latissimus dorsi flap, musculofascial flap, or other pedicles. The further development of these strategies will help to improve the outcome of synthetic-based trachea because of the enhanced integrity of the graft and ameliorated in situ regeneration of the transplant.

The pros of this method are that it is not donor dependent, there is no need for immunosuppressive medication, it is anatomically tailored, processing is fast and low-cost, and the nature of its mechanical properties. The cons are that the material is nonvital and there is a risk for contamination.

Composite scaffolds

Biologic and synthetic materials can also be combined into one scaffold to optimize the mechanical and bioactive properties of the graft. The coating of artificial scaffolds with various natural ligands and ECM-proteins may enhance cell adherence and proliferation while mechanical forces maintain. Research has been performed on collagen-coated poly-propylene scaffolds. In addition, various gels incorporating the cells for the internal and external surface were investigated.[40] The outcome of all these surface modification studies did not result in entirely convincing data; therefore, clinical transfer has not been realized.[41,42] In contrast, defects of the trachea smaller than 50 mm, have been successfully treated with the technology of composites using a Marlex mesh tube covered by collagen sponge.[43] Therefore, combinations of biologic and synthetic components may provide novel alternatives to TE in the future. The pros of this method are that it is not donor dependent, there is no need for immunosuppressive medication, it can be customized, and processing is fast, and cost-effective. The cons are that it is stent-dependent, nonvital, and there is a risk for contamination.

Scaffold-free

A recently developed technology of scaffold-free cell sheets is so far only applicable for very small defects but not for circumferential defects or longer gap reconstructions due to the lack of structural integrity.

The pros are that this method is not donor dependent and there is no need for immunosuppressive medication. The cons are that it is not feasible for long gap and circumferential reconstruction.

Cells

The cell type and source can differ and is highly dependent on the target tissue (**Fig. 1**). Considerations include stem versus differentiated cells, and allogenic versus autologous cells.

Aside from in vitro seeded cells, bone marrow-derived cells and resident stem or progenitor cells may contribute to tissue regeneration.[44] Go and colleagues,[45] and Jungebluth and colleagues,[38] demonstrated the necessity of seeding cells before tracheal transplantation to avoid graft collapse and bacterial contamination. Seguin and colleagues[44] provided similar evidence for the involvement of bone marrow–derived mesenchymal stem cells to tracheal regeneration. In addition, resident stem and progenitor cells, responsible for tissue regeneration and repair, have been detected in so-called stem cell niches along the airways, so far mainly in animals but similarities may exist in humans.[46,47]

Stem cells

Pluripotent stem cells The use of pluripotent cells, including embryonic stem cells (ESCs) and induced pluripotent stem cells (iPSCs) is widely debated. In particular, ESCs are controversial because of significant ethical concerns. When Takahashi and Yamanaka[48] first described the technology of reprogramming mature cells into pluripotent stem cells, it was presumed that this cell type would soon be transferred to the clinic and be an ideal autologous alternative to ESCs. However, in experimental studies it has been elucidated that both iPSCs (depending on the reprogramming method) and ESCs seem to be prone to immune recognition and consequent rejection. In addition, the reprogramming for IPSCs is insufficient, which makes clinical use currently unrealistic. The pros of pluripotent cells are that they are not donor dependent (iPSCs) and there is no need for immunosuppressive medication (method dependent). The cons are ethical concerns, donor dependency (ESCs), and the need for immunosuppressive medication.

Multipotent stem cells Multipotent or adult stem cells, such as mesenchymal (MSCs), hematopoietic stem cells (HSCs), or amniotic fluid stem cells,

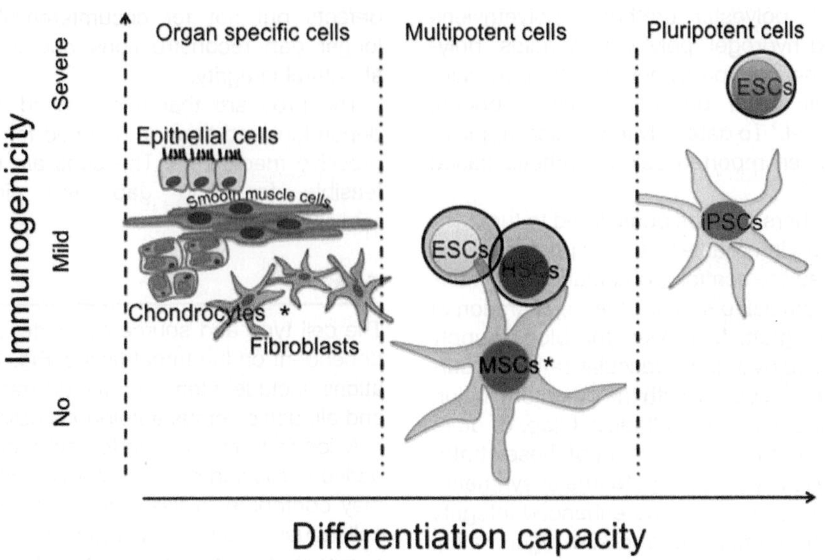

Fig. 1. Immunogenicity of various cell types potentially usable in TE. EPCs, endothelial progenitor cells; ESCs, embryonic stem cells; HSCs, hematopoietic stem cells; iPSCs, induced pluripotent stem cells; MSC, mesenchymal stromal cells. Already clinically applied (*asterisks*).

can differentiate into various cell types. These stem cells are usually obtained from the recipient (eg, bone marrow, peripheral blood, fat tissue) with essentially no ethical concerns and, therefore, can be applied without the use of immunosuppression. These so-called adult stem cells have already been used in many tracheal-related and nonrelated clinical settings.[27,49–51] Mononuclear cells (MNCs) have become clinically interesting (NCT01110252) because they include stem and progenitor cells, can be isolated from the bone marrow or the peripheral blood, and be actively mobilized to increase the yield of isolated cells.[37]

The pros of this method are there is no need for immunosuppressive medication, it is not donor dependent (depending on the cell type), multipotent differentiation, good availability, immunomodulatory capacity, and nearly no ethical issues. The con is that it is donor dependent.

Terminally differentiated cells

Epithelial, smooth muscle, and endothelial cells, and chondrocytes, have been clinically applied[14,27,32,35] for different tracheal replacement strategies. All these cells have low ethical implications, which make the clinical transfer simple.

The pros for this method are no need for immunosuppressive medication (depending on cell source), it is not donor dependent (if autologous), and isolation is simple. The cons are that it is donor dependent (if allogenic), immunosuppression (for allogenic) is needed, it is terminally differentiated, and the cell numbers are low.

Autologous versus allogenic cells

The advantage of using autologous cells is that it eliminates the patient's need for lifelong immunesuppressants. Regarding adult stem and progenitor cells, the available number and application field are high because of their self-renewal and differentiation capacity. In contrast, terminally differentiated cells have a limited source due to autologous cell or tissue donations making them inappropriate for some specific clinical scenarios. Allogenic cells have an unlimited availability but, aside from MSCs, require lifelong immunosuppressive medication.

The pros of allogenic cells are the unlimited cells numbers and the capacity for differentiation depending on the cell type. The cons are the need for immunosuppressive medication (except for MSCs). The pros of autologous cells are that they are not donor dependent and no immunosuppressive medication is needed. The cons are limited cell numbers and that they are inappropriate for malignant diseases (see **Fig. 1**).

Bioreactor

To provide the ideal conditions for TE of the airways, the natural environment should be ideally mimicked or used as a bioreactor. The external conditions influence all cellular parameters such as adhesion, engraftment, proliferation, differentiation, migration, and apoptosis. Asnaghi and colleagues[52] introduced a double-chamber rotating bioreactor for trachea engineering in a clinical setting with controlled and monitored conditions.

A more developed version of this bioreactor has been used for the clinical transplantation of natural decellularized scaffolds[27,34] and synthetic-based grafts.[37,38] Despite these initial promising clinical applications, there is the possibility of using the organism of the organ recipient as a biologic bioreactor with an single-[53,54] or multistage in vivo engineering strategy.[14]

In vitro pros are controlled and monitored conditions and customized devices. The cons are risk of contamination, lack of native characteristics, the need for additional substrates (eg, hormones, growth factors), cost, and labor demands.

In vivo pros are an ideal environment and it is cost-effective. The con is that there is no control of cell behavior (proliferation, migration, differentiation).

Pharmaceutical Intervention

Bioactive and signaling molecules, hormones, and other factors may be used to overcome the difficulties associated to engineered tissue transplantation, especially contamination and, even more significant, necrosis. Vascularization or, more precisely, neovascularization plays the most crucial role in this context and usually results in ischemia of the transplanted tissue. Direct and indirect vascularization can be achieved via surgical techniques as previously described.[11] However, additional strategies are necessary to provide sufficient angiogenesis within the transplanted construct. Therefore, other vascular growth promoting factors are required, such as vascular endothelial growth factor, fibroblast growth factor, and so forth. Aside from the bioactive factors that drive the neovascularization, further components such as endothelial cells are necessary to form the novel vessels. To this end, strategies that can mobilize progenitor and stem cells from their niches are of interest (**Fig. 2**), including granulocyte colony-stimulating factor (G-CSF), which was administrated in some early patients who underwent tracheal transplantation.[37] G-CSF can mobilize endothelial progenitor cells (EPCs) to support neoangiogenesis and MSCs can positively influence wound healing. MSCs, specifically CXCR-4–positive MSCs, can be attracted to the transplantation site and promote the regeneration of the implanted graft via their immunomodulatory capacity. The cell homing is initiated and driven by various blood activation products, chemokines, and/or growths factors and can be mediated through the SDF-1/CXCR4 pathway. Usually, an ischemic environment dominates the surgical wound due to initially poorly developed

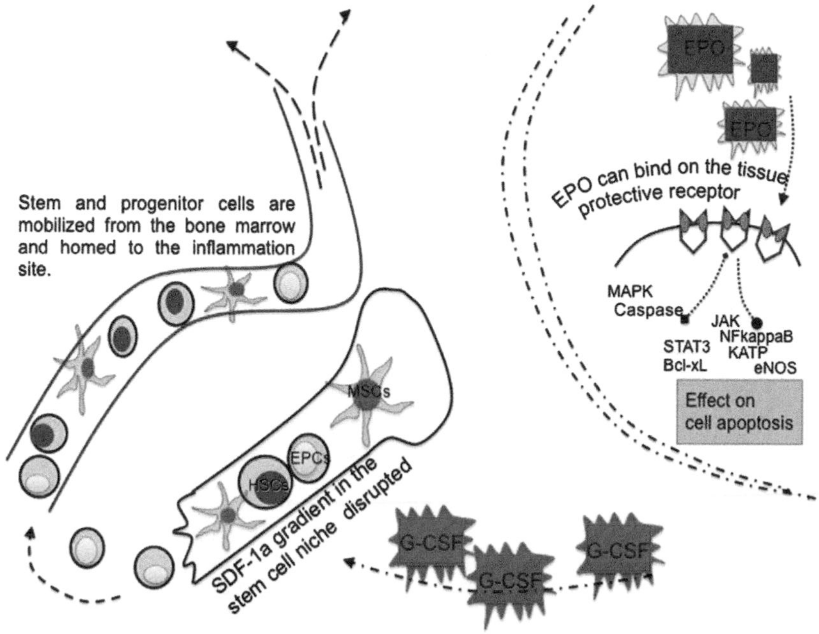

Fig. 2. Pharmaceutical intervention and bioactive molecules. EPCs, endothelial progenitor cells; EPO, erythropoietin; G-CSF, granulocyte colony-stimulating factor; HSCs, hematopoietic stem cells. Genes involved in apoptosis: Bcl-xL, B-cell lymphoma-extra large; eNOS, endothelial nitric oxide synthase; JAK, Janus kinase; KATP, ATP-sensitive K(+); MAPK, mitogen-activated protein kinases; MSC, mesenchymal stromal cells; NFkappaB, nuclear factor kappa-light-chain-enhancer of activated B cells; STAT3, signal transducer and activator of transcription 3.

neovascularization, which provokes increased cell death. Antiapoptotic strategies, therefore, may have beneficial impact on transplanted tissues. Erythropoietin (EPO) can certainly represent such a tool via its tissue protective function that has been described previously.[55,56] Aside from regulating the erythropoiesis, EPO influences the expression of several antiapoptotic genes, including Janus tyrosine kinase-2 (JAK-2) STAT5 (signal transducer and activator of transcription 5)-Bcl-2, phosphatidylinositol 3, protein kinase B, mitogen-activated protein kinase, and nuclear factor-κB. Using EPO may provide a protective effect for resident cells (within the wound environment) and to cells that are exposed to ischemic environment on the tracheal graft due to the lack of early vascularization.

Further strategies focus on the modification of the scaffold to improve cell–surface interaction and the material's biocompatibility and, therefore, the cell adhesion, proliferation, and differentiation. The pro of this method is support of the endogenous regenerative capacity. The cons are unknown risks and side-effects.

SUMMARY

Trachea transplantation remains a highly challenging procedure and, so far, no ultimate solution has been discovered. For many decades, physicians and researchers made immense efforts to overcome the hurdles of replacing a simple connection between the larynx and the lungs. It turned out to be much more difficult and, in particular, more complex than previously assumed. Various purely surgical techniques have been evaluated; however, because of technical challenges, they have not proven their clinical feasibility. In addition, conventional allogenic transplantation requires lifelong immunosuppressive medication and is associated with negative side effects. Recently, early clinical achievements in tissue-engineered trachea provide clinical evidence that this method might be the next promising therapeutic alternative in tracheal replacement (**Table 3**). Progress has been made in investigating underlying mechanisms and pathways of cell–surface interactions, cell migration, and differentiation; however, we are far from fully understanding the complexity of tracheal tissue regeneration. TE is

Table 3
Overview of clinical cases using TE tracheal grafts

	Decellularized Trachea Transplantation (2008–2011)	**Outcome**
Patients	9 male/female (3:6) (11–72 y)	4:5 (dead/alive)
Indications		
Benign diseases (n = 6)	4	All 4 alive, partly biodegradable stent-dependent
• Severe tracheomalacia or bronchomalacia	1	Alive, no need for stent support
• Long-segment congenital stenosis	1	Patient died of fulminant gastrointestinal bleeding
• Tracheoesophageal fistula		
Malignant diseases (n = 3)	3	All patients died of systemic tumor recurrence
• Primary tracheal carcinoma		
	Synthetic-based Trachea (2011–2013)	**Outcome**
Patients	Eight male/female, 3:5 (2–43 y)	2:6 (dead/alive)
Indications		
Benign diseases (n = 6)		1 (out of 6) patient died of unrelated causes
• Severe tracheomalacia or bronchomalacia	4	To date, all patients are alive (only the POSS/PCU scaffold requires stent treatment because of abnormal granulation tissue and fistula formation)
• Long-segment congenital stenosis	1	
• Congenital agenesis	1	
Malignant diseases (n = 2)	2	1 patient died of severe gastrointestinal bleeding
• Primary tracheal carcinoma		

a step in the right direction but only the future will elucidate the real impact of this technology on tracheal replacement.

REFERENCES

1. Grillo HC. Tracheal replacement: a critical review. Ann Thorac Surg 2002;73:1995–2004.
2. Nakahira M, Nakatani H, Takeuchi S, et al. Safe reconstruction of a large cervico-mediastinal tracheal defect with a pectoralis major myocutaneous flap and free costal cartilage grafts. Auris Nasus Larynx 2006;33:203–6.
3. Macchiarini P. Primary tracheal tumours. Lancet Oncol 2006;7:83–91.
4. Fonkalsrud EW, Sumida S. Tracheal replacement with autologous esophagus for tracheal stricture. Arch Surg 1971;102:139–42.
5. Fonkalsrud EW, Martelle RR, Maloney JV. Surgical treatment of tracheal agenesis. J Thorac Cardiovasc Surg 1963;45:520–5.
6. Rose K, Sesterhenn K, Wustrow F. Tracheal allotransplantation in man. Lancet 1979;1:433.
7. Levashov Yu N, Yablonsky PK, Cherny SM, et al. One-stage allotransplantation of thoracic segment of the trachea in a patient with idiopathic fibrosing mediastinitis and marked tracheal stenosis. Eur J Cardiothorac Surg 1993;7:383–6.
8. Delaere PR, Liu Z, Sciot R, et al. The role of immunosuppression in the long-term survival of tracheal allografts. Arch Otolaryngol Head Neck Surg 1996;122:1201–8.
9. Shaari CM, Farber D, Brandwein MS, et al. Characterizing the antigenic profile of the human trachea: implications for tracheal transplantation. Head Neck 1998;20:522–7.
10. Klepetko W, Marta GM, Wisser W, et al. Heterotopic tracheal transplantation with omentum wrapping in the abdominal position preserves functional and structural integrity of a human tracheal allograft. J Thorac Cardiovasc Surg 2004;127:862–7.
11. Macchiarini P, Lenot B, De Montpreville V, et al. Heterotopic pig model for direct revascularization and venous drainage of tracheal allografts. Paris-Sud University Lung Transplantation Group. J Thorac Cardiovasc Surg 1994;108:1066–75.
12. Duque E, Duque J, Nieves M, et al. Management of larynx and trachea donors. Transplant Proc 2007;39:2076–8.
13. Farwell DG, Birchall MA, Macchiarini P, et al. Laryngotracheal transplantation: technical modifications and functional outcomes. Laryngoscope 2013;123(10):2502–8. http://dx.doi.org/10.1002/lary.24053.
14. Delaere P, Vranckx J, Verleden G, et al. Tracheal allotransplantation after withdrawal of immunosuppressive therapy. N Engl J Med 2010;362:138–45.
15. Kunachak S, Kulapaditharom B, Vajaradul Y, et al. Cryopreserved, irradiated tracheal homograft transplantation for laryngotracheal reconstruction in human beings. Otolaryngol Head Neck Surg 2000;122:911–6.
16. Yokomise H, Inui K, Wada H, et al. High-dose irradiation prevents rejection of canine tracheal allografts. J Thorac Cardiovasc Surg 1994;107:1391–7.
17. Liu Y, Nakamura T, Sekine T, et al. New type of tracheal bioartificial organ treated with detergent: maintaining cartilage viability is necessary for successful immunosuppressant free allotransplantation. ASAIO J 2002;48:21–5.
18. Hisamatsu C, Maeda K, Tanaka H, et al. Transplantation of the cryopreserved tracheal allograft in growing rabbits: effect of immunosuppressant. Pediatr Surg Int 2006;22:881–5.
19. Jacobs JP, Quintessenza JA, Andrews T, et al. Tracheal allograft reconstruction: the total North American and worldwide pediatric experiences. Ann Thorac Surg 1999;68:1043–51 [discussion: 1052].
20. Elliott MJ, Haw MP, Jacobs JP, et al. Tracheal reconstruction in children using cadaveric homograft trachea. Eur J Cardiothorac Surg 1996;10:707–12.
21. Carbognani P, Spaggiari L, Solli P, et al. Experimental tracheal transplantation using a cryopreserved aortic allograft. Eur Surg Res 1999;31:210–5.
22. Wurtz A, Porte H, Conti M, et al. Tracheal replacement with aortic allografts. N Engl J Med 2006;355:1938–40.
23. Wurtz A, Porte H, Conti M, et al. Surgical technique and results of tracheal and carinal replacement with aortic allografts for salivary gland-type carcinoma. J Thorac Cardiovasc Surg 2010;140:387–93.e2.
24. Wurtz A, Hysi I, Kipnis E, et al. Tracheal reconstruction with a composite graft: fascial flap-wrapped allogenic aorta with external cartilage-ring support. Interact Cardiovasc Thorac Surg 2013;16:37–43.
25. Olausson M, Patil PB, Kuna VK, et al. Transplantation of an allogeneic vein bioengineered with autologous stem cells: a proof-of-concept study. Lancet 2012;6736:1–8.
26. Atala A, Bauer SB, Soker S, et al. Tissue-engineered autologous bladders for patients needing cystoplasty. Lancet 2006;367:1241–6.
27. Macchiarini P, Jungebluth P, Go T, et al. Clinical transplantation of a tissue-engineered airway. Lancet 2008;372:2023–30.
28. Cebotari S, Lichtenberg A, Tudorache I, et al. Clinical application of tissue engineered human heart valves using autologous progenitor cells. Circulation 2006;114:I132–7.
29. Jungebluth P, Go T, Asnaghi A, et al. Structural and morphologic evaluation of a novel

detergent-enzymatic tissue-engineered tracheal tubular matrix. J Thorac Cardiovasc Surg 2009; 138:586–93 [discussion: 592–3].
30. Conconi MT, DeCoppi P, Di Liddo R, et al. Tracheal matrices, obtained by a detergent-enzymatic method, support in vitro the adhesion of chondrocytes and tracheal epithelial cells. Transpl Int 2005;18:727–34.
31. Zang M, Zhang Q, Chang EI, et al. Decellularized tracheal matrix scaffold for tissue engineering. Plast Reconstr Surg 2012;130:532–40.
32. Walles T, Giere B, Hofmann M, et al. Experimental generation of a tissue-engineered functional and vascularized trachea. J Thorac Cardiovasc Surg 2004;128:900–6.
33. Seguin A, Radu D, Holder-Espinasse M, et al. Tracheal replacement with cryopreserved, decellularized, or glutaraldehyde-treated aortic allografts. Ann Thorac Surg 2009;87:861–7.
34. Elliott MJ, De Coppi P, Speggiorin S, et al. Stem-cell-based, tissue engineered tracheal replacement in a child: a 2-year follow-up study. Lancet 2012;380:994–1000.
35. Macchiarini P, Walles T, Biancosino C, et al. First human transplantation of a bioengineered airway tissue. J Thorac Cardiovasc Surg 2004;128:638–41.
36. Macchiarini P. La transplantation de trachée et trachéo-oesophagienne [Thesis]. Berançon (France): Université Franche-Comte; 1997.
37. Jungebluth P, Alici E, Baiguera S, et al. Tracheobronchial transplantation with a stem-cell-seeded bioartificial nanocomposite: a proof-of-concept study. Lancet 2011;378:1997–2004.
38. Jungebluth P, Haag JC, Lim ML, et al. Verification of cell viability in bioengineered tissues and organs before clinical transplantation. Biomaterials 2013; 34:4057–67.
39. Available at: http://www.nytimes.com/2013/04/30/science/groundbreaking-surgery-for-girl-born-without-windpipe.html?_r=0.
40. Tada Y, Suzuki T, Takezawa T, et al. Regeneration of tracheal epithelium utilizing a novel bipotential collagen scaffold. Ann Otol Rhinol Laryngol 2008; 117:359–65.
41. Yanagi M, Kishida A, Shimotakahara T, et al. Experimental study of bioactive polyurethane sponge as an artificial trachea. ASAIO J 1994;40:M412–8.
42. Grimmer JF, Gunnlaugsson CB, Alsberg E, et al. Tracheal reconstruction using tissue-engineered cartilage. Arch Otolaryngol Head Neck Surg 2004;130:1191–6.
43. Omori K, Tada Y, Suzuki T, et al. Clinical application of in situ tissue engineering using a scaffolding technique for reconstruction of the larynx and trachea. Ann Otol Rhinol Laryngol 2008;117:673–8.
44. Seguin A, Baccari S, Holder-Espinasse M, et al. Tracheal regeneration: evidence of bone marrow mesenchymal stem cell involvement. J Thorac Cardiovasc Surg 2013;145(5):1297–304.e2. http://dx.doi.org/10.1016/j.jtcvs.2012.09.079.
45. Go T, Jungebluth P, Baiguero S, et al. Both epithelial cells and mesenchymal stem cell-derived chondrocytes contribute to the survival of tissue-engineered airway transplants in pigs. J Thorac Cardiovasc Surg 2010;139:437–43.
46. Kim CF, Jackson EL, Woolfenden AE, et al. Identification of bronchioalveolar stem cells in normal lung and lung cancer. Cell 2005;121:823–35.
47. Reya T, Morrison SJ, Clarke MF, et al. Stem cells, cancer, and cancer stem cells. Nature 2001;414: 105–11.
48. Takahashi K, Yamanaka S. Induction of pluripotent stem cells from mouse embryonic and adult fibroblast cultures by defined factors. Cell 2006;126: 663–76.
49. Gupta PK, Chullikana A, Parakh R, et al. A double blind randomized placebo controlled phase I/II study assessing the safety and efficacy of allogeneic bone marrow derived mesenchymal stem cell in critical limb ischemia. J Transl Med 2013; 11:143.
50. Miettinen JA, Salonen RJ, Ylitalo K, et al. The effect of bone marrow microenvironment on the functional properties of the therapeutic bone marrow-derived cells in patients with acute myocardial infarction. J Transl Med 2012;10:66.
51. Le Blanc K, Frassoni F, Ball L, et al. Mesenchymal stem cells for treatment of steroid-resistant, severe, acute graft-versus-host disease: a phase II study. Lancet 2008;371:1579–86.
52. Asnaghi MA, Jungebluth P, Raimondi MT, et al. A double-chamber rotating bioreactor for the development of tissue-engineered hollow organs: from concept to clinical trial. Biomaterials 2009; 30:5260–9.
53. Bader A, Macchiarini P. Moving towards in situ tracheal regeneration: the bionic tissue engineered transplantation approach. J Cell Mol Med 2010;14: 1877–89.
54. Jungebluth P, Bader A, Baiguera S, et al. The concept of in vivo airway tissue engineering. Biomaterials 2012;33:4319–26.
55. Brines M, Cerami A. Erythropoietin-mediated tissue protection: reducing collateral damage from the primary injury response. J Intern Med 2008;264:405–32.
56. Hoch M, Fischer P, Stapel B, et al. Erythropoietin preserves the endothelial differentiation capacity of cardiac progenitor cells and reduces heart failure during anticancer therapies. Cell Stem Cell 2011;9:131–43.

Management of Tracheal Surgery Complications

Gunda Leschber

KEYWORDS

• Tracheal surgery complications • Granuloma • Dehiscence • Restenosis
• Tracheo-innominate artery fistula

KEY POINTS

- There are several factors influencing the success of tracheal operations and the rate of complications.
- Besides risk factors on the part of the patient, such as prior tracheal surgery, tracheostomy tube in place, extent and localization of the tracheal disease, and need for release maneuvers, the experience of the surgeon also plays a major role in preventing complications.
- Good clinical judgment, careful planning of the procedure, and meticulous dissection as well as knowledge of salvage maneuvers will result in a low complication rate in tracheal surgery.
- The learning curve of tracheal surgery includes intraoperative experience and dealing with postoperative complications.
- Often observing further healing ("wait and see") instead of premature action will result in good outcome.

INTRODUCTION

Tracheal surgery in general is only rarely complicated by undesired effects; however, if complications occur, they can lead to severe morbidity.[1–3] Several factors influence the outcome after tracheal surgery, such as reoperations, preoperative tracheostomy, diabetes, pediatric patients, or the length of the resected segment.[1]

Prevention of complications starts preoperatively with treatment of acute infectious or inflammatory conditions.[4] A noninflamed mucosa is optimal for surgery and there is seldom a need for rushing an operative procedure.[2]

Intraoperative complications are extremely infrequent if the operative team is familiar with airway surgery (ie, surgeon, anesthetist, and assisting personnel), because there is a learning curve.[3,5] Management of intubation (via bronchoscopy or over the operative field) and handling of extended resections with release maneuvers do not pose a problem for an experienced team. Some postoperative complications however originate from intraoperative manipulation. These complications are anastomotic granulations, stenosis, or anastomotic dehiscence as well as bleeding from vessel arrosion. Other complications include injuries of recurrent laryngeal nerve, arrhythmias, pneumonia, or wound infection.

PREVALENCE OF POSTOPERATIVE COMPLICATIONS IN TRACHEAL SURGERY

The most complete analysis of anastomotic complications after tracheal operation was presented in 2004 by Wright and colleagues[1] from the Massachusetts General Hospital (MGH). In their review of 901 patients they identified relevant risk factors and described the management of problems. Anastomotic complications included granulations at the suture line, stenosis, and tracheal separation. A good result at the end of treatment was

Disclosure: None.
Department of Thoracic Surgery, ELK Berlin Chest Hospital, Lindenberger Weg 27, Berlin 13125, Germany
E-mail address: gunda.leschber@elk-berlin.de

Thorac Surg Clin 24 (2014) 107–116
http://dx.doi.org/10.1016/j.thorsurg.2013.09.002
1547-4127/14/$ – see front matter

seen in 95% of patients with no need for a tracheostomy tube or T-tube (**Table 1**). Four percent of patients needed a permanent airway appliance, and mortality was 1.2%. They analyzed different indications of airway surgery and their complication rate (postintubation stenosis, tracheoesophageal fistula, laryngotracheal stenosis, and tumor). Overall complications were observed most frequently in the tracheoesophageal fistula group (28.6%) with anastomotic complications in 14.3% because this is the most complex group with often a tracheostomy in place (which is considered an independent risk factor because it renders the operative field infectious). The fewest problems with the anastomosis (2.4%) were seen in the laryngotracheal stenosis group for a total complication rate of 6.6% in this group. Eighty-one patients (9%) experienced anastomotic complications in their series: 37 patients had dehiscence, 7 had granulation with airway obstruction, and 37 developed stenosis. Treatment included multiple dilations (n = 2), temporary tracheostomy (n = 7), tracheal T-tube (n = 16), permanent tracheostomy (n = 14), or T-tube (n = 20) as well as reoperation (n = 16). If anastomotic complications occurred, mortality was 7.4% (6/81) compared with 0.06% (5/820) in those without anastomotic problems. Since 1988 no patients died, which is attributed to the routine use of postoperative bronchoscopy for early recognition a problems. They also described a significant reduction in suture granuloma formation since the conversion to absorbable suture material.

Wright and colleagues identified several predictors of anastomotic complications: reoperation, preoperative tracheostomy, lengthy (>4 cm) resections, and the need for a release maneuver. Other predictors of anastomotic complications were diabetes, age less than 17 years, and laryngotracheal resections (**Table 2**). The release maneuver itself was not considered an independent risk factor because it only indicated the need for extensive resection. Neither obesity nor corticosteroid use was associated with an increased complication rate. Management strategy is to postpone tracheal operations in the presence of high-dose steroids until they are effectively tapered.

D'Andrilli and coworkers[6] summarized complications from multiple studies in laryngotracheal resections for benign stenosis (**Table 3**). Again, success rates were greater than 91%. In their own group over a period of 16 years (with a mean follow-up of 61 months) they observed a restenosis rate of 11.4%. These patients were successfully treated by endoscopic interventions with final success of 100%. Friedel and coworkers[7] evaluated the long-term results of 110 tracheal segmental resections performed between 1985 and 2001. Again, healing of the anastomosis was uncomplicated in 91.8% (101 patients) and complication rates were according to what is described in the literature. They interviewed 77 patients for the long-term results 12 to 226 months postoperatively (median 80.1 months): 93.5% (n = 72) were satisfied with the surgical treatment, 75.3% were without discomfort, 9.1% reported stridor when exercising, and 11.7% complained of occasional hoarseness. Three patients required reoperation for restenosis because of suture dehiscence, foreign body granuloma, and localized recurrence of mucoepidermoid carcinoma. Only 6.5% (5 patients) were not satisfied with the results of surgery because of persistent hoarseness and stridor under exercise.

Table 1
Anastomotic complications after tracheal resection: results of MGH

	Total	PITS	Tumor	ILTS	TEF
Number of cases	901	589	206	83	21
Complication (%)	18.2	18.5	19.7	6.6	28.6
Dehiscence (%)	9.0	11.0	5.3	2.4	14.3
Mortality (%)	1.2	1.4	1.0	0	4.8
Good result (%)	95.0	95.2	97.1	98.8	90.0
Tracheal cannula (%)	4.2	4.8	2.9	1.2	10.0

Abbreviations: ILTS, idiopathic laryngotracheal stenosis; PITS, postintubation tracheal stenosis; TEF, tracheoesophageal fistula.

Adapted from Wright CD, Grillo HC, Wain JC, et al. Anastomotic complications after tracheal resection: prognostic factors and management. J Thorac Cardiovasc Surg 2004;128(5):733; with permission.

PREVENTION OF COMPLICATIONS IN TRACHEAL SURGERY

To achieve low complication rates in tracheal surgery, it is important to have a concept of protective strategy before operating.

Exact Planning of Operative Procedure

Before operation, the cause and location of the tracheal disease should be fully understood, so the surgeon can exactly plan the operative procedure and thereby reduce probable complications. Tracheal surgery, more than other operations, warrants an interdisciplinary approach whereby it is important to have competent partners, not only anesthetists but also otolaryngologists and bronchoscopists, if necessary. Besides the "how-to-do-it" also the timing of the operation or necessary

Table 2
Predictors of anastomotic complications resection: results of MGH

	No Separation (91%, n = 820)	Separation (9%, n = 81)	Univariable Odds Ratio	95% Confidence Interval	*P* Value
Reoperation (%)	9.4	29.6	4.06	2.39–6.91	<.0001
Preoperative tracheostomy (%)	28.3	54.3	3.01	1.89–4.79	<.0001
Length ≥4 cm (%)	29	50.6	2.51	1.58–3.97	<.0001
Length ± SD (cm)	3.25 ± 0.9	3.72 ± 1.1	1.61	1.28–2.02	.0005
Release (%)	7.2	27.2	4.81	2.76–8.39	<.0001
Age ≤17 y (%)	6	16	3.0	1.56–5.82	.0006
Diabetes (%)	9.5	22.2	2.72	1.53–4.82	.0004
Laryngotracheal resection (%)	30.2	40.7	1.59	0.99–2.53	.05

Adapted from Wright CD, Grillo HC, Wain JC, et al. Anastomotic complications after tracheal resection: prognostic factors and management. J Thorac Cardiovasc Surg 2004;128(5):733; with permission.

preoperative preparations are best discussed together to achieve optimal results.

Knowledge of Patient's History

It is important to be familiar with the history of the disease, prior surgical attempts, or the placement of a tracheostomy tube. Corticosteroids should be terminated or tapered as much as possible before surgery because they are responsible for adverse wound-healing effects.

Knowledge of Radiological Findings

A posteroanterior chest radiograph may reveal some tracheal pathologic abnormality. However, the standard now is high-resolution computed tomographic (CT) scan with 3-dimensional reconstruction. It allows determination of the extraluminal component of underlying pathologic abnormality in the case of malignant disease or the longitudinal extension of the stenosis (**Fig. 1**).

Bronchoscopy by the Surgeon

Bronchoscopy is the key element to confirm the diagnosis and plan the operative strategy. Either a rigid or a flexible scope can be used to measure the length of stenosis as well as the length of normal trachea available, both proximal and distal to the pathologic abnormality. It can also identify the anatomic relations, cricoid, and first tracheal ring (**Fig. 2**).

Table 3
Complications in laryngotracheal resections in benign stenosis

		Results						
Author (year)	Pts	Successes (%)	Failures (%)	Restenosis (%)	Compl. (%)	Mortality (%)	Reop (%)	Dehiscence (%)
Grillo, 1995	62	92	8	5.5[a]	33	2.4	3.4	5.5[a]
Couraud, 1995	57	98.2	1.8	0	3.5	1.8	0	1.8
Macchiarini, 2001	45	96	4	4.4	41	2	2.2	0
Ashiku, 2004	73	91	9	8.3	8.2	0	0	0
D'Andrilli, 2008	35	Early: 85.7 Definitive: 100	Early: 14.3 Definitive: 0	11.4	11.3	0	0	2.9

[a] Restenoses + dehiscences.
Data from D'Andrilli A, Rendina EA, Venuta F. Tracheal surgery. Monaldi Arch Chest Dis 2010;73(3):108.

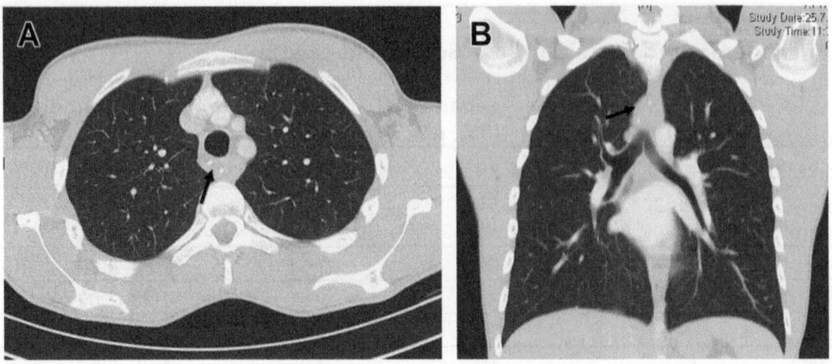

Fig. 1. (*A, B*) CT scan of a tumor with calcifications (*black arrow*), located behind the trachea.

Treatment of Mucosal Inflammation or Tracheobronchial Infection

In the case of mucosal inflammation or ulcerations, surgery should be delayed until mucosal healing occurs. If this is due to a tracheostomy tube, it may require a change to a smaller tube or if possibly even a short period of decannulation. In patients with idiopathic laryngotracheal stenosis with active inflammation an attempt of dilatation is indicated until the inflammatory state of the airway mucosa subsides. Tracheobronchial infections should be treated preoperatively according to the microbiologic evaluation to achieve optimal condition for surgery.

Intraoperative Measures for Prevention of Complications

Intraoperatively handling of the trachea should be as gentle as possible, which can be difficult in tense adhesions and scar tissue from previous operations. Staying close to the tracheal wall avoids impairment of the recurrent laryngeal nerve or laceration of the esophagus. The use of pinpoint bipolar coagulation in the vicinity of trachea and nerve also prevents damage. Denudation from the adjacent tissue must be avoided to keep blood supply intact. If the trachea at the distal end of the stenosis is incised transversally, the ventral part of the stenosis can be opened, allowing resection of the stenosis under direct vision and freeing of the posterior wall as well.

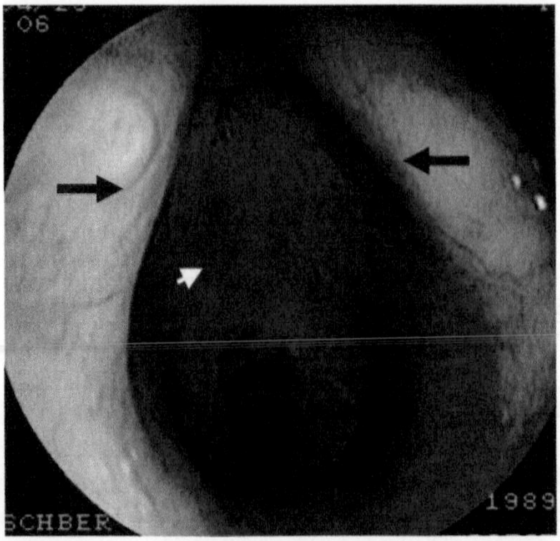

Fig. 2. Preoperative bronchoscopy: anatomic relation of a localized stenosis in the upper trachea: note the vocal cords (*black arrows*) and cricoid (*white arrowhead*). The mucosa shows signs of inflammation.

Approximation of the cut ends for the anastomosis is facilitated by stay sutures in the cranial and caudal parts, which are held by the assistant; also flexion of the neck when the sutures are tied decreased tension at the suture line. Extubation at the end of the operative procedure is good protection from further disturbances of mucosal blood flow and should be done whenever possible.

Postoperative Care

Good aftercare is essential to patients who have undergone tracheal operations because respiratory difficulties may require immediate intervention. Patients should be observed in the intensive care unit for signs of swelling of the anastomosis or bleeding and for phonation and swallowing. If immediate extubation was not possible, weaning from mechanical ventilation should be attempted as soon as possible.

Patients should have their neck in anteflexion with a pillow all the times for at least 5 days and avoid brisk movements of the head. In the author's experience, it is not necessary to use any chin-to-chest-stitches.

COMPLICATION MANAGEMENT DURING THE TRACHEAL RESECTION

Problems with Ventilation

At induction of anesthesia problems may occur. An experienced anesthetist and the surgeon should be available as well as (rigid) bronchoscopes of different sizes. Bronchoscopic dilatation before intubation allows insertion of an endotracheal tube larger than expected from the stenosis. In fixed stenosis, impossible to be dilated, only a small endotracheal tube can be placed distally to the obstructive lesion. In the rare event that ventilation cannot be installed, an emergency transverse incision of the trachea and intubation over the operative field will save the patient's life. Intraoperatively a cross-field intubation may become necessary if jet ventilation fails to achieve sufficient oxygenation or elimination of CO_2.

Tension of Anastomosis

While completing the tracheal anastomosis, tension should be kept to a minimum. Until now the only way to judge anastomotic tension is experience because no viable method exists to determine constant tension. A short residual trachea increases the tension of the anastomosis. If this is only minor, a long additional stay suture between tracheal rings above and below the anastomosis on the anterior part of the trachea can be placed to reduce anastomotic tension. However, surgeons performing tracheal surgery must be familiar with release maneuvers, which are indicated in cases with short residual trachea (ie, mobilization of the larynx, the main bronchi, or pericardial incision; see Hecker and colleagues in this issue). Flexing the neck anteriorly lowers the tension while performing the anastomosis. Postoperatively the patient needs to keep the neck flexed for at least a week. One simple method described in the literature is to sew the lower jaw to the anterior chest wall with a suture. However, in the author's experience as well as others,[7] an extra pillow is sufficient to assure anteflexion in cooperative patients.

Bleeding

During resection of the diseased segment of the trachea, meticulous hemostasis is indicated. Bleeding from the peritracheal tissue or the mucosa can cause annoyance during formation of the anastomosis. The use of bipolar forceps is very helpful to stop bleeding from the mucosa because of its efficiency and limitation of damage, especially close to the recurrent laryngeal nerve.

Resection of Wrong Trachea Level

Reference to preoperative bronchoscopy (level of the diseased part in relation to cricoid or the bifurcation) and CT will enable the experienced surgeon to define the exact level of resection. Intraoperatively thyroid, cricoid, and carina are anatomic landmarks for positioning but extensive scar tissue may obscure orientation in some cases. Then, intraoperative bronchoscopy for localization of the lesion should be performed by the anesthetist while the surgeon inserts a needle through the tracheal wall to define the level of disease. Exploring the extent of the stenosis under direct vision can be performed if the ventral tracheal wall is opened.

These tricks should avoid resection of the wrong trachea height. If, however, a false level is resected, further mobilization of the trachea (ie, with release maneuvers) is indicated.

Level of Stenosis is Higher than Expected

If intraoperatively found that the level of stenosis extends higher than preoperatively expected, a cricotracheal resection may be indicated. It may be sufficient to perform a Pearson procedure,[8] or an additional Montgomery suprahyoid release of the larynx may be necessary to gain an additional 1.5 cm of length[9]; these are release maneuvers effective for achieving additional mobility of the cervical trachea.

MANAGEMENT OF POSTOPERATIVE COMPLICATIONS

Bleeding Caused by Tracheo-innominate Artery Fistula

Bleeding within the first 2 days postoperatively is more likely due to venous injury of the inferior thyroid or the anterior jugular veins. In contrast, formation of a tracheo-innominate artery fistula is a rare complication (0.1%–1%).[10] An ongoing infection at the site of the anastomosis or a tracheostomy tube is cause for the formation of a such a fistula, which explains why this occurs generally within the first 3 weeks postoperatively (72% of cases).[11]

In about 50% a herald bleed precedes the massive hemorrhage so, if de novo minor bleeding from the tracheal tube or the surrounding structures is observed, immediate investigation should be initiated. One should be prepared to maintain the airway with an endotracheal tube and have suction available to remove blood from the oropharynx or trachea if a sentinel bleed is suspected. A bronchoscopy (flexible and/or rigid) should be performed in the operating room with careful removal of the tracheostomy tube. Because of the anatomic relation, the injury most likely occurs at the level of the seventh to nineth tracheal ring but with the variability of the innominate artery (brachiocephalic artery) it can occur also at higher levels of the trachea.

If a massive hemorrhage occurs from the trachea, the initial goal is to control the airway by endotracheal intubation. At the same time an attempt to tamponade the bleeding should be undertaken while the patient is resuscitated and prepared for surgery. Compression of the tracheo-innominate artery fistula by overinflating the tracheal cuff as a first maneuver can be successful.[12] If not, blunt finger dissection of the pretracheal space should be performed down to the level of the innominate artery after widening the tracheostomy incision. The innominate artery can then be pressed against the posterior sternum to control the bleeding (**Fig. 3**).

When the diagnosis of tracheo-innominate artery fistula is clear on presentation, the patient should be intubated immediately with the endotracheal tube inserted distally and the balloon inflated for prevention of bleeding into the distal airway for expeditious transportation to the operating room. Manual compression of the fistula should be attempted.

Operative Management

Median sternotomy provides the best exposure and is expedient. However, it can result in postoperative mediastinitis because of the infectious origin of the tracheo-innominate artery fistula (studies describe up to 40%).[10] As soon as the innominate artery (brachiocephalic artery) is identified, it is clamped proximally and distally (**Fig. 4**). (It may be necessary to mobilize and divide the innominate vein first.) The involved part is resected and the healthy proximal and distal ends of the innominate artery are stapled, oversewn, or ligated (**Fig. 5**).[13] The incidence of stroke is low after such a maneuver but care should be taken to ligate the artery proximally to the bifurcation of the right subclavian and common carotid arteries. Because of the division of the innominate artery one should have a left radial arterial line in place for blood pressure monitoring and a large-bore venous access in the femoral or right subclavian veins because of possible innominate vein ligation.

There is a controversy about immediate reconstruction of the innominate artery because of the high risk of recurrent bleeding (60%–86%).[11] However, in the presence of severe left carotid artery stenosis/occlusion or a patent right internal mammary artery bypass graft, this could be considered. The interposition is done by a vein graft (saphenous or jugular vein). It is not recommended to perform a segmental resection and primary repair of the artery (without interposition) because tension seems to be too high with a risk of recurrent bleeding.

Sorial and coworkers[14] in 2007 described successful percutaneous stent graft insertion for control of an acute hemorrhage in infected operative

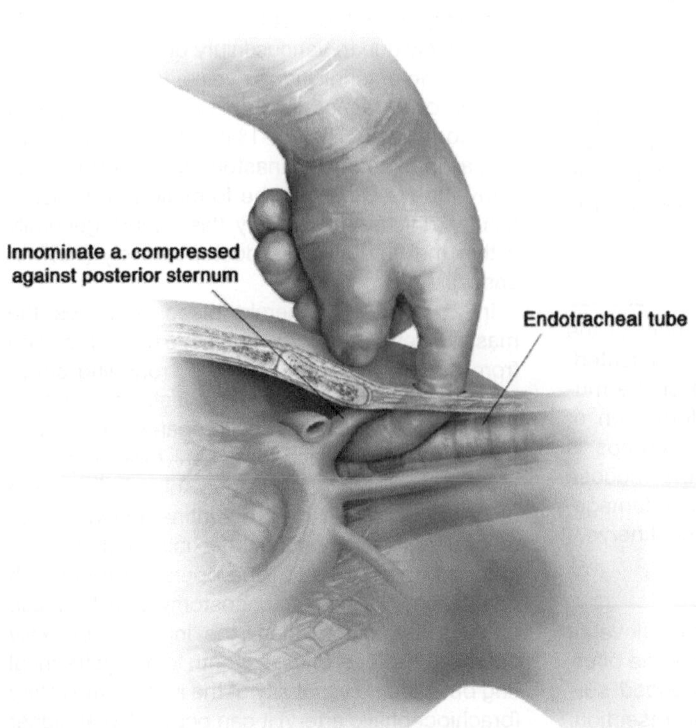

Fig. 3. Digital compression of innominate artery against the sternum. a., artery. (*From* Ailawadi G. Technique for managing tracheo-innominate artery fistula. Oper Tech Thorac Cardiovasc Surg 2009;14:68. Copyright 2009; with permission.)

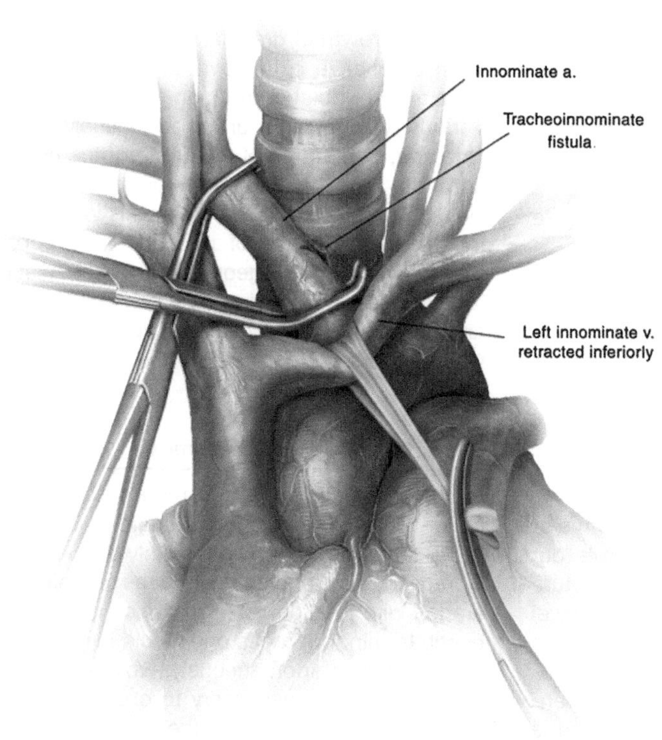

Fig. 4. Clamping of innominate artery proximal and distal to the fistula. a., artery; v., vein. (*From* Ailawadi G. Technique for managing tracheoinnominate artery fistula. Oper Tech Thorac Cardiovasc Surg 2009;14:69. Copyright 2009; with permission.)

fields as a bridging procedure. Depending on the status of the patient, debridement and reconstruction of the innominate artery can be performed at a later date.

Following separation of the artery, the tracheal lesion is debrided up to the healthy part and then repaired with interrupted sutures. For additional securing of the tracheal wound or separation of

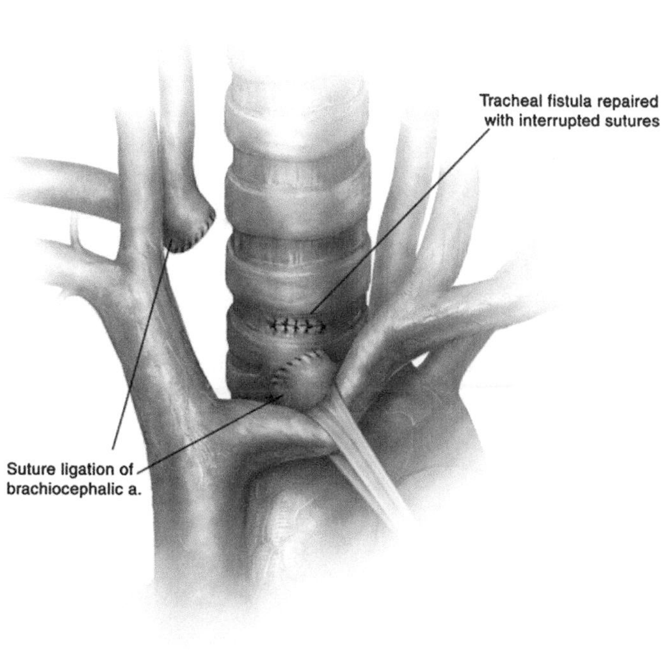

Fig. 5. Suturing of innominate artery and trachea. a., artery. (*From* Ailawadi G. Technique for managing tracheo-innominate artery fistula. Oper Tech Thorac Cardiovasc Surg 2009;14:70. Copyright 2009; with permission.)

trachea and innominate artery, a muscle flap using the sternocleidomastoideus or strap muscles is buttressed to the trachea (**Fig. 6**). Sashida and Arashiro[15] described an anatomic reconstruction by a synthetic graft in combination with a pectoralis muscle flap.

Granuloma Formation at the Anastomotic Site

A certain degree of intraluminal granulation at the anastomotic site is seen frequently after tracheal surgery in the postoperative phase without any need for intervention. It should be controlled by bronchoscopy because in most cases it will resolve spontaneously. It is important to refrain from unnecessary interventions! Patience on the part of the surgeon is often the key to success (**Fig. 7**).

However, if a more distinct granuloma forms at the anastomosis, bronchoscopy should rule out that this is due to loose sutures. Sometimes suture material creates a permanent irritation at the level of the mucosa and by removing these sutures granuloma will resolve by itself. The use of absorbable sutures has decreased the incidence of granuloma formation.[1,7] Another presumed reason is some degree of separation of the anastomosis, allowing ingrowth of granulation tissue.[1]

An alternative of removal of persistent granuloma is laser ablation through the bronchoscope. Various types of laser are used routinely in medicine and, depending of the depth of the coagulation, the laser type should be chosen.[16] The Nd:YAG laser is widely used for this indication as the maximum depth of penetration is approximately 4 mm. The surgeon or bronchoscopist performing the laser ablation must be familiar with the anatomy and the laser to remove the granuloma without doing further harm to the anastomosis or mucosa.

Dehiscence of the Anastomosis

Anastomotic dehiscence, a more severe complication, can occur in different degrees. It presents either as partial separation, mainly of the cartilaginous part of the anastomosis, or as complete separation with total dehiscence, which is a dramatic event. In minor degrees one would just observe if healing occurs spontaneously, which is often the case.[7] It may be necessary to open the cervical wound to drain a peritracheal abscess, which

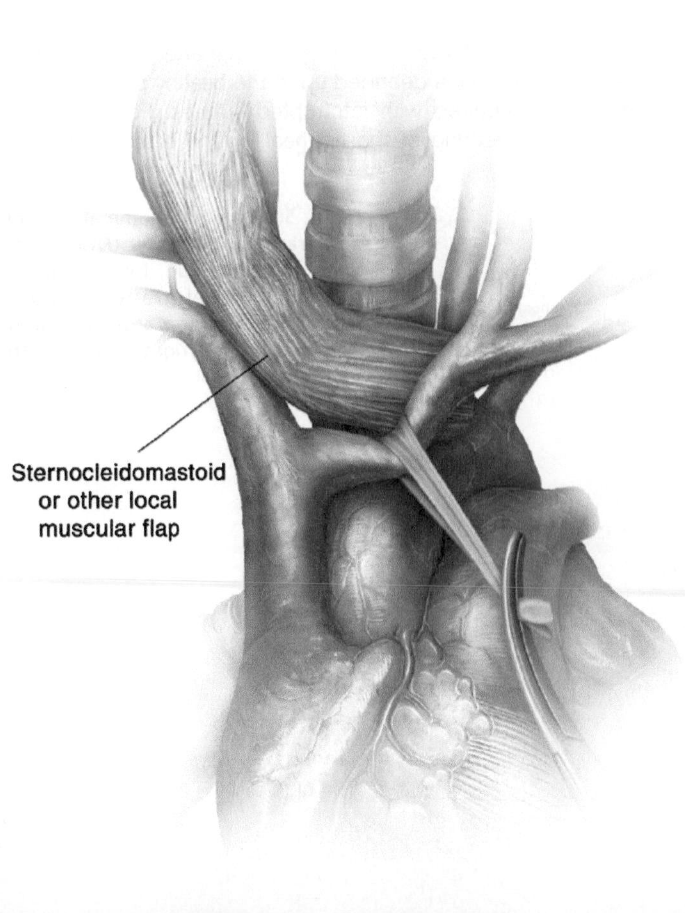

Fig. 6. Buttressing of the muscle to the trachea. (*From* Ailawadi G. Technique for managing tracheo-innominate artery fistula. Oper Tech Thorac Cardiovasc Surg 2009;14:66–72. Copyright 2009; with permission.)

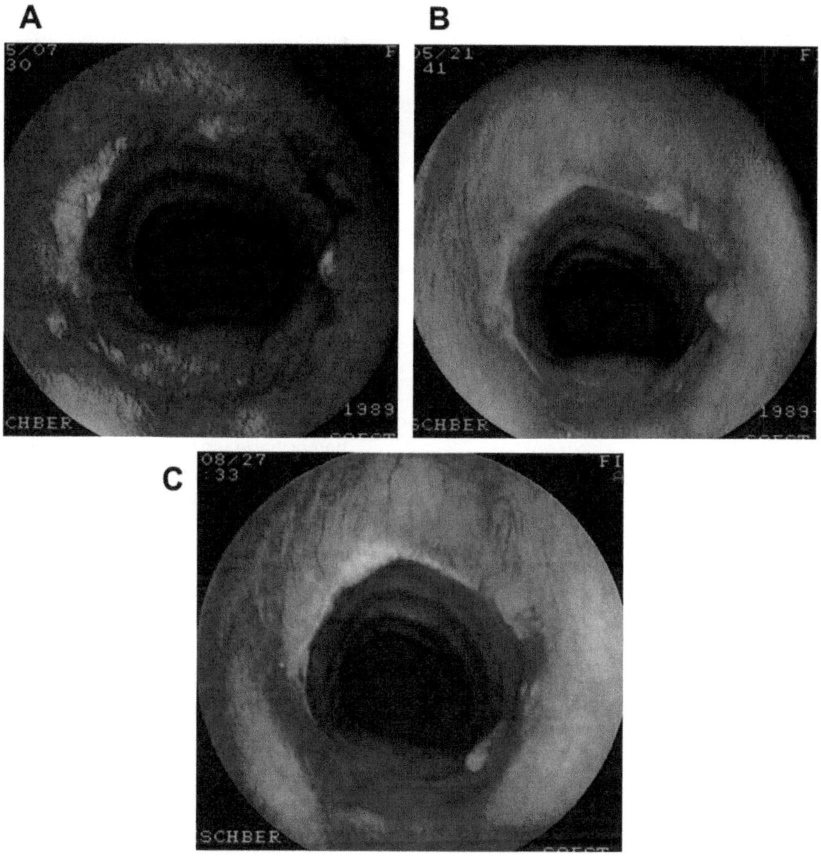

Fig. 7. (*A–C*) Resolution of granuloma at the anastomotic site following resection of a tracheal stenosis (same patient as in **Fig. 2**). (*A*) 10 d postoperatively. (*B*) 1 month postoperatively. (*C*) 3 months postoperatively.

caused the partial dehiscence.[2] Repeat bronchoscopy is performed to assess if a more severe dehiscence develops. Then, insertion of a t-tube is indicated; in rare cases an attempt to reoperate can be made. Placement of stent can be discussed but because of the already impaired blood supply of the tracheal wall additional pressure by a stent may further deteriorate the healing process.

Restenosis

If restenosis occurs, management will be the same as for primary stenosis (ie, evaluation for reoperation, laser therapy, and stent or tracheostomy placement). Depending on the time point of development of a restenosis, the method should be chosen. An early restenosis is an indication for insufficient resection of the primary disease and may be cured by reoperation by a more experienced tracheal surgeon. However, most restenoses develop over a longer period of time. Both granulations and dehiscence can lead to an anastomotic stenosis, which can also be caused by insufficient perfusion of the tracheal wall. Patients should be informed about the risks of redo procedures.

CONCLUSION

In conclusion, there are several factors influencing the success of tracheal operations and the rate of complications. Besides risk factors from the patient, such as prior tracheal surgery, tracheostomy tube in place, extent and localization of the tracheal disease, and need for release maneuvers, the experience of the surgeon also plays a major role in preventing complications. Good clinical judgment, careful planning of the procedure, and meticulous dissection as well as knowledge of salvage maneuvers results in a low complication rates in tracheal surgery. The learning curve of tracheal surgery has been described by many authors[3,5]: this includes intraoperative experience and dealing with postoperative complications. Often observing further healing ("wait and see") instead of premature action will result in a good outcome.

REFERENCES

1. Wright CD, Grillo HC, Wain JC, et al. Anastomotic complications after tracheal resection: prognostic

factors and management. J Thorac Cardiovasc Surg 2004;128(5):731–9.
2. Engelmann C. Chirurgisch relevante Trachealäsionen bei Erwachsenen und ihre Therapie. Z Herz-, Thorax-. Gefäßchir 1995;9:125–37.
3. Grillo HC, Zannini P, Michealssi F. Complications of tracheal reconstruction. Incidence, treatment and prevention. J Thorac Cardiovasc Surg 1986;91: 322–8.
4. Krajc T, Janik M, Lucenic M, et al. The managment of restonosis following segmental resection for postintubation tracheal injury. Rozhl Chir 2010; 89(8):490–7.
5. Mansour KA, Lee RB, Miller JI Jr. Tracheal resctions: lessons learned. Ann Thorac Surg 1994; 57(5):1120–4.
6. D'Andrilli A, Rendina EA, Venuta F. Tracheal surgery. Monaldi Arch Chest Dis 2010;73(3):105–15.
7. Friedel G, Kyriss T, Leitenberger A, et al. Long-term results after 110 tracheal resections. Ger Med Sci 2003;1. Doc10 online.
8. Pearson FG, Cooper JD, Nelems JM, et al. Primary tracheal anastomosis after resection of the cricoid cartilage with preservation of recurrent laryngeal nerves. J Thorac Cardiovasc Surg 1975;70:806–16.
9. Montgomery WW. Suprahyoid release for tracheal anastomosis. Arch Otolaryngol 1974;99:225–60.
10. Allan JS, Wright CD. Tracheoinnominate fistula: diagnosis and management. Chest Surg Clin N Am 2003;13(2):331–41.
11. Gellman JJ, Aro M, Weiss SM. Tracheo-innominate artery fistula. J Am Coll Surg 1994;179(5):624–34.
12. Ailawadi G. Technique for managing tracheo-innominate artery fistula. Operat Tech Thorac Cardiovasc Surg 2009;14:66–72.
13. Ridley RW, Zwischenberger JB. Tracheoinnominate fistula: surgical management of an iatrogenic disaster. J Laryngol Otol 2006;120(8):676–80.
14. Sorial E, Valentino J, Given CA, et al. The emergency use of endografts in the carotid circulation to control hemorrhage in potentially contaminated fields. J Vasc Surg 2007;46(4):792–8.
15. Sashida Y, Arashiro K. Successful management of tracheoinnominate artery fistula using a split pectoralis muscle flap with anatomical reconstruction by synthetic graft. Scand J Plast Reconstr Surg Hand Surg 2010;44(3):175–7.
16. Dumon JF, Reboud E, Garbe L, et al. Treatment of tracheobronchial lesions by laser photoresection. Chest 1982;81(3):278–84.

Treatment of Malignant Tracheoesophageal Fistula

Martin Hürtgen[a], Sascha C.A. Herber[b,*]

KEYWORDS

• Tracheoesophageal fistula • Enterorespiratory fistula • Endobronchial stenting
• Endoesophageal stenting • Interventional bronchoscopy • Interventional esophagoscopy
• Interventional radiology

KEY POINTS

- This article focuses on the interventional treatment of malignant enterorespiratory fistulas, especially tracheoesophageal fistula (TEF).
- TEF is a devastating condition for the patient, and typically occurs after radiochemotherapy for advanced esophageal cancer or extensive mediastinal nodal disease from lung cancer.
- Life expectancy of these patients is measured in months after successful treatment of the fistula, and only days to weeks with a persistent fistula.
- To stop repeated episodes of aspiration and septic pneumonia, single or double stenting of the esophagus and trachea with self-expandable coated stents is the established palliative treatment.
- Surgical interventions are justified only in very select cases, and carry a very high morbidity and mortality.

INTRODUCTION

Fistulas from the enteric tract to the respiratory tract can develop in more ways than as a tracheoesophageal fistula (TEF).[1] As the abbreviation TEF is often used to refer also to fistulas between the stomach and bronchi or lung, this context is used for TEF in this article. Because benign TEF has been dealt with extensively in a previous issue of this series,[2] the authors concentrate here on malignant TEF (mTEF), and describe in detail modern palliative treatment options and their typical problems.

The issues and interventions in benign fistulas are markedly different. Typically the fistula develops in a patient with other major medical issues, often as a complication of prolonged intubation. Many, if not most of these fistulas can be approached surgically with a relatively small operation using a cervical approach. Repair of the fistula is often difficult, but with interposition of healthy tissue (eg, strap muscle, sternocleidomastoid or pectoralis muscle) and removal/repositioning of the inciting cause of the fistula (ie, tracheostomy tube, nasogastric tube), good results can be obtained if the patient is able to recover from the underlying major medical problem. Stenting often aggravates the problem, and long-term complications (granulation tissue, dried secretions) make this a less appealing long-term solution. In patients without life-threatening comorbidities, a substernal gastric bypass can offer long-term functional ability to eat without aspiration through the fistula.

EPIDEMIOLOGY OF MTEF

TEF develops in approximately 5% to 15% of patients with an esophageal malignancy and in less than 1% of those with bronchogenic carcinoma.[3–5] Most patients with mTEF suffer from esophageal cancer and very few from other

[a] Thoracic Surgery Department, Catholic Clinics Koblenz-Montabaur, University Teaching Hospital, R. Virchow Street 7, 56073 Koblenz, Germany; [b] Radiology Department, Catholic Clinics Koblenz-Montabaur, University Teaching Hospital, R. Virchow Street 7, 56073 Koblenz, Germany
* Corresponding author.
E-mail address: s.herber@kk-km.de

Thorac Surg Clin 24 (2014) 117–127
http://dx.doi.org/10.1016/j.thorsurg.2013.09.006

malignancies: 19 of 264 (7.2%) pulmonary tumors and 2 of 264 (0.8%) mediastinal tumors in the series from Balazs and colleagues.[5] The incidence of mTEF seems to have increased over the last 30 years to a level well above 10% of all nonresected esophageal cancers. Malignant TEF usually develops during or after completing radiochemotherapy for tumor necrosis in an area that previously showed tumor progression into the wall of the tracheobronchial system. The fistula site is esophagotracheal in 52% to 57% of patients and esophagobronchial in 37% to 40%. In the remaining patients (3%–11%), communication is established peripherally, through the lung parenchyma, forming an esophagopulmonary fistula.[6] The attribution of development of mTEF to necrosis induced by radiochemotherapy is controversial in the literature and is not statistically confirmed. Balazs and colleagues[5] found only 4 of their 264 cases to have developed TEF within 4 weeks of beginning radiation therapy, and suggest that TEF is more frequently observed after radiation therapy because of the prolonged survival observed with radiochemotherapy.

SYMPTOMS AND DIAGNOSIS

Typical symptoms of mTEF, such as coughing, aspiration, and pneumonia, are neither uncommon nor surprising during radiochemotherapy. Thus the recognition of the formation of TEF may be delayed for 1 to 18 months after the first clinical symptoms.[5] Patients may present in severe septic condition, with manifest aspiration pneumonia as the most frequent symptom (95% in the study of Balazs and colleagues[5]). Clinical confirmation of TEF is most easily achieved using a swallowing test of water in the presence of an experienced doctor. Water-soluble contrast swallowed under fluoroscopic control can achieve definitive diagnosis, estimation of the size, and exact topographic description of TEF (**Fig. 1**). Additional computed tomography (CT) scanning immediately after swallowing contrast media can give further information about the location of the TEF relative to areas of tumor necrosis, may show deposits of contrast media in the mediastinum, and is helpful for planning further treatment. Endoscopic confirmation of the esophageal fistula opening is mostly easy, as it is the larger orifice of both fistula endings. In smaller fistulas, recognition of the tracheal or bronchial opening (**Fig. 2**) can be challenging and requires some experience.

TREATMENT

Because of the underlying disease and radiation therapy, the general condition of these patients is always severely deteriorated. Repeated episodes

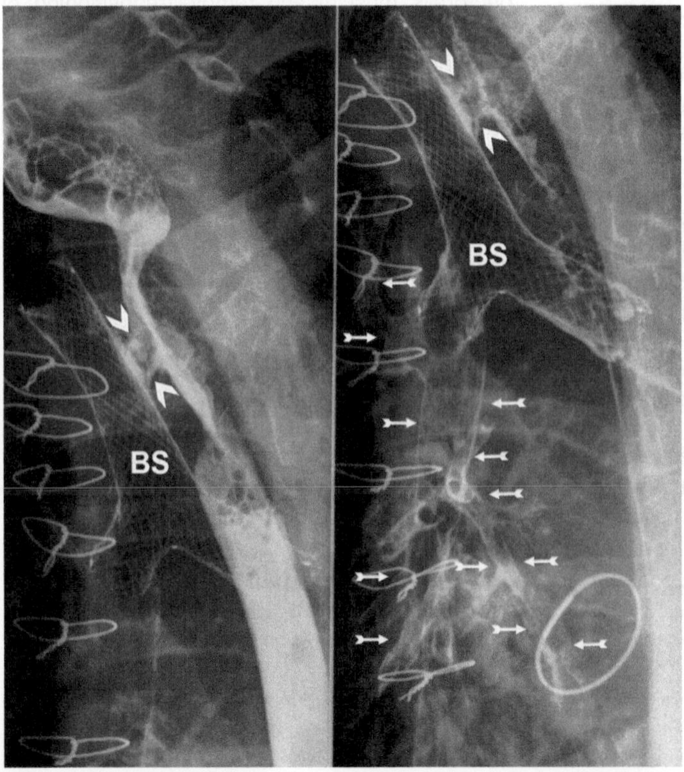

Fig. 1. Persisting tracheoesophageal fistula (TEF) (*arrowheads*) after positioning a bronchial Y-stent (BS), with leakage along the stent and "bronchography" (*arrows*) by the aspiration of contrast media, illustrating why primary esophageal stenting is preferable and mere stenting of the trachea frequently is insufficient.

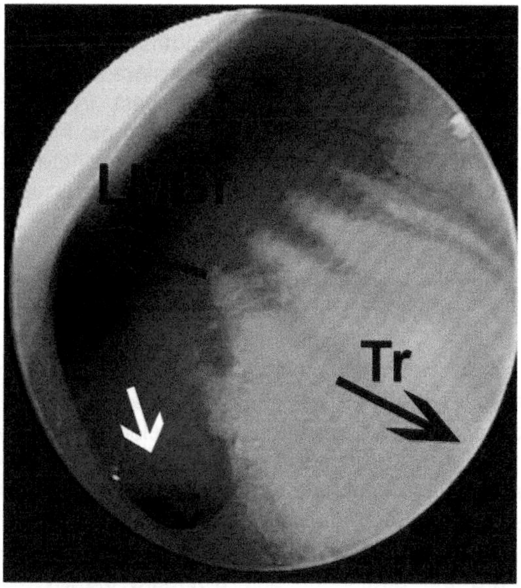

Fig. 2. TEF (*white arrow*) at the origin of the left main bronchus (LMBr); wires of the esophageal stent can be seen at the bottom of the fistula. Tr, trachea.

of aspiration pneumonia can lead to respiratory insufficiency. Remaining life expectancy is measured in weeks to months. In this situation, major surgery for esophageal exclusion and extra-anatomical reconstruction of the gastrointestinal passage is rarely a reasonable option, whereas rapid and minimally invasive closure of the fistula, to stop repeated aspiration, is of utmost importance. Since the introduction of covered self-expanding stents, reports on the surgical treatment of TEF with esophageal bypass surgery have been episodic,[7] and such an extensive and potentially complicated procedure in a patient with only few months left to live may be justified in very select cases only. Davydov and colleagues[1] tried esophagectomy in 35 TEF patients, resulting in a complication rate of 40% and a mortality rate of 14.3%; this was the price for the comparably long median survival of 13 months (range 3–31 months) and a 2-year survival rate of 21% in the selected subgroup of patients who did survive the procedure.

Nowadays in countries with a well-developed medical system and established interdisciplinary cooperation, for the aforementioned reasons the treatment of mTEF is predominantly interventional and not surgical.

Esophageal Stenting

It is logical to attempt closing the esophageal fistula orifice first, after taking into account the natural direction of any aspirate from the esophageal lumen into the respiratory system. In many cases this is sufficient to stop the clinical symptoms of TEF. Stenting TEF in the esophagus does not differ much from primary stenting of esophageal cancer, besides which sometimes a stenosis is missed to help secure the position of the stent. Paradoxically, stenosis is helpful in esophageal stenting, as it prevents the stent from dislocation.

Basically, the technique of esophageal stenting using an endoscopic or radiologic approach is very similar. In fact, the endoscopist will advance the guide wire through the stenosis under visual control and then proceed under fluoroscopic visualization exactly as the radiologist would. The radiologist may be familiar with more techniques with which to manage very narrow stenosis or even occlusions. Radiologic equipment such as wires and guiding catheters are distinctly thinner than the typical endoscopic material, and allow passage through a high-grade stenosis in most cases. The interventional procedure is undertaken ideally on a dedicated C-arm angiography unit. In difficult cases, the opportunity to enlarge the display window and to rotate the image amplifier might be the key to depict critical details and to ensure the passage through the stenosis without complication. Nevertheless, use of a less advanced fluoroscopy unit might be feasible.

Nowadays, coated self-expanding metallic (typically nitinol) stents or plastic stents are typically chosen. Stents are coated with a membrane (eg, polyethylene, silicone) to avoid tumor invasion and to safely cover the fistula site. Depending on the extent of this membrane, one can differentiate between fully and partially covered stents. Before any interventional treatment, a radiographic examination of the esophagus (with isoosmolar or hypo-osmolar water-soluble radiograph contrast medium) (see **Fig. 1**) is recommended for exact localization of the fistula and for treatment planning. Based on the radiographic images, stent length and diameter can be determined. The stent should cover at least 2 cm of healthy esophageal wall, proximal and distal to the fistula margins, and be wide enough to press firmly against the esophageal wall. Unfortunately, these dimensions are not always possible, or they provoke secondary problems depending on the level of the TEF. In very high proximal TEF, the stent cannot sit higher than the upper esophageal sphincter, and therefore will not sufficiently seal to the esophageal wall. Furthermore, in higher fistulas a very wide stent might compress the adjacent trachea in the narrow upper mediastinum. In addition to different stent lengths, a variety of stent types are available. Covered stents tend to dislocate more than uncovered stents, because the coating prevents the imbedding of the device into the esophageal wall. To avoid stent displacement, so-called flared-ended stents are now widely used. At their proximal and distal end, these stents are 4 to 6 mm larger in diameter than the body of the stent. The progressive flared ends may reduce the risk of stent migration.

For esophageal stenting, analgosedation, for example with midazolam or propofol combined with a morphine derivative (eg, piritramide or pethidine), is safe and sufficient in most cases. However, cardiorespiratory surveillance is strongly advised. After local anesthesia of the oral cavity (eg, with lidocaine spray) the hypopharynx and upper esophageal sphincter are passed using the flexible endoscope, or directly with a hydrophilic guide wire (0.035 in [0.089 cm]), and a 4F to 5F guiding catheter. In the endoscopic approach, if the tumor region can be easily passed by the endoscope, or at least the lumen is endoscopically visible, the guide wire can be introduced directly through the working channel of the scope, which is withdrawn afterward. In cases of subtotal stenosis or complete occlusion, the guiding catheter is placed directly proximal to the closure. After this, isoosmolar or hypoosmolar water-soluble contrast medium is administered. If the passage of contrast media is still possible, the guide wire is advanced through the constriction and placed safely, distally to the TEF. In rare cases of complete esophageal occlusion with TEF, careful probing with the soft tip of the guide wire, supported by a rigid guiding catheter that gives enough stability for the procedure, might lead to passage through the problem zone. In difficult and desperate cases, a combined antegrade and retrograde access with probing of the stomach and transgastral access to the esophagus should be considered.

After successful passage of the TEF, the guide wire and the guiding catheter are advanced until the distal esophagus or the stomach is reached. A stiff J-tip guide wire should then be inserted over the primarily placed guiding catheter. Compared with soft wire, the stiff wire provides a much better support for the passage of a very tight and rigid stenosis, and avoids dislocation of the device.

Modern stent devices have an outer diameter of 6.0 to 8.0 mm. In cases with severe stenosis, or even occlusion, primary passage by the introducer device may be impossible. In such cases balloon dilatation is carried out first. The balloon is inserted using the "over-the-wire technique" via the already placed guide wire. The use of a noncompliable high-pressure balloon catheter (eg, 8.0–12.0 mm balloon diameter) is standard. After correct placement of the balloon markers, the balloon is slowly inflated with a diluted water-soluble contrast medium until the hourglass deformity created by the stricture disappears from the balloon contour. The authors recommend the use of a manometer syringe, which may facilitate the opening of sometimes very rigid strictures and provides a reliable pressure control.

After repeated fluoroscopic examination and documentation of the correct guide-wire position, the self-expanding stent is advanced over the super-stiff wire (**Fig. 3**A). For the stent deployment, the fistula first is passed with almost two-thirds of the stent body. Most stents are released from the distal end. The stent primarily is released slightly distal to the intended final position. Self-expanding stents tend to dislocate forward or shorten in a dilated esophagus. In addition, in high-grade stenosis the stent may be "sucked" toward the bottleneck and dislocate distally. To avoid this uncontrolled jumping of the stent, the authors first only open it partially, after which the stent may be retracted under fluoroscopic visual control and then fully deployed in the target area. This method prevents an imperfect stent placement in most cases. In fact, it is much easier to pull the stent backward than to push it distally. Because of their strong radial force, self-expanding metal stents will further expand in the 48 to 72 hours following stent deployment, and postplacement stent dilatation should be considered restrictively.

The patient is remitted to the ward, and after 2 to 3 hours is allowed to sip some water. The following day the stent position and expansion is checked, and the elimination of the TEF is documented with an additional radiographic examination using orally administered contrast medium.

In cases with a typical prestenotic dilatation of the esophagus, a leakage of contrast medium might persist around the proximal stent ending (**Fig. 4**) between the stent body and the esophageal wall that maintains the fistula. This problem is well known in the elimination of vessel aneurysms and is called endoleakage. The problem may be solved by the extension of the stenting more proximally in the region of a "normal" esophagus diameter, as performed by Saxon and colleagues.[8] Other attempts at closure with injection of tissue glue reported by Wang and colleagues[9] and Devière and colleagues[10] were less successful.

Airway stenosis and persistent leakage along the esophageal stent are indications for secondary tracheobronchial stenting. To prevent stridor after esophageal stenting, everything should be prepared for intubating the patient temporarily so

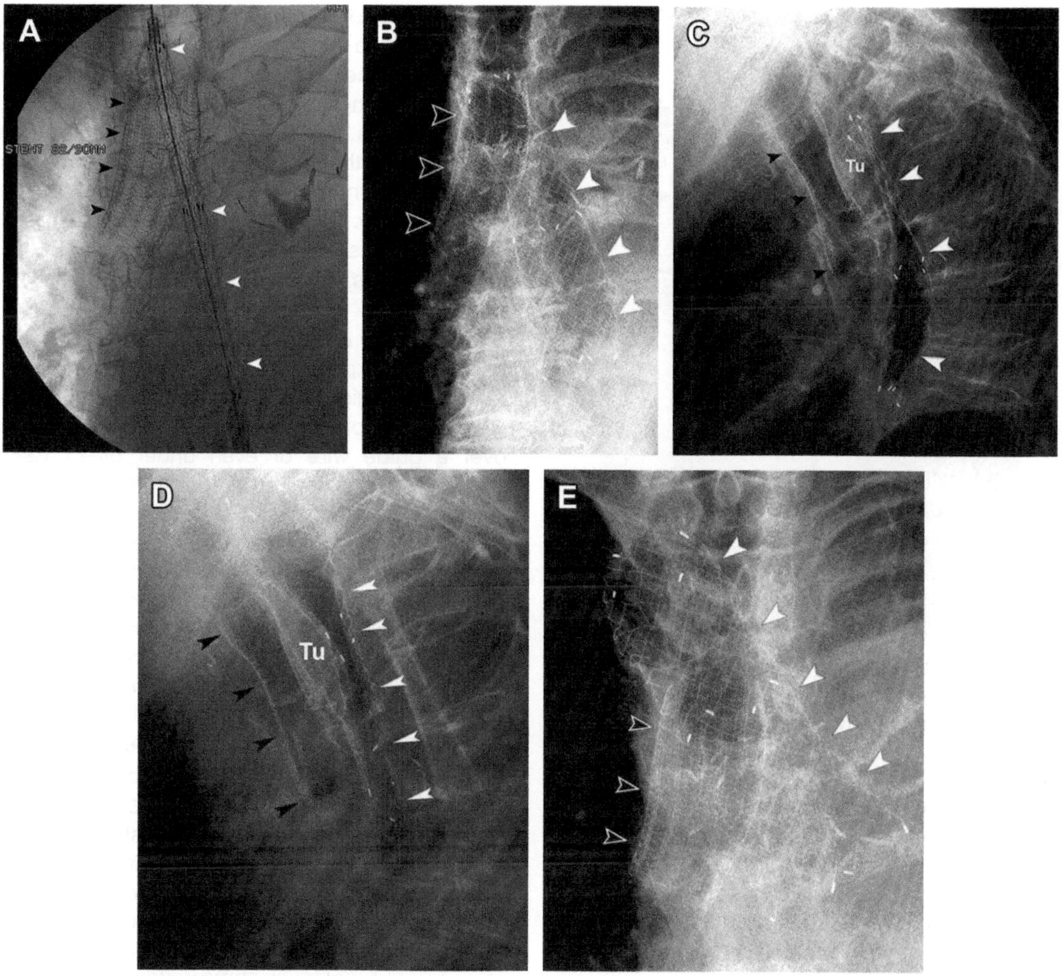

Fig. 3. (*A*) Double stenting. On secondary stenting of the esophagus, the tracheal stent (*black arrowheads*) is already in situ, and the esophageal stent (*white arrowheads*) is just about to be deployed. (*B*) Double stenting. Radiograph of both stents in posteroanterior projection appears regular at a first glance (*arrowheads* as in *A*). (*C*) Radiograph of both stents in lateral projection shows collapse of the proximal part of the esophageal stent owing to compression from tumor and tracheal stent (*arrowheads* as in *A*). Tu, tumor compressing esophagus and trachea. (*D*) Same radiograph projection as in *C*. The esophageal stent has been pulled back to a more oral position, which allows full expansion of the esophageal stent's proximal part (*arrowheads* as in *A*). (*E*) Same situation as *D*, but with posteroanterior projection (*arrowheads* as in *A*).

as to continue with tracheal stenting as soon as possible.

Tracheobronchoscopic Stenting

Respiratory management during interventional bronchoscopy in patients with an open TEF is demanding, and requires that pulmonary infections be managed first. Antibiotics, and correction of dehydration and electrolyte imbalance by intravenous infusions, are usually required before bronchoscopic stenting.

The gastroenterologist may ask the pneumologist or thoracic surgeon for tracheal stenting, even before esophageal stenting, in a case that seems untreatable with esophageal stenting, or because he or she fears compressing the trachea significantly with the esophageal stent. This reasoning also explains why all 5 patients in the study of Chen and colleagues[4] received airway stenting first. The authors prefer esophageal stenting first, and proceed with tracheal stenting only if unavoidable, because of typical secondary problems of double stenting (see **Fig. 3**C).

Anesthesiologic peri-interventional management

The following points about peri-interventional management should be considered very carefully

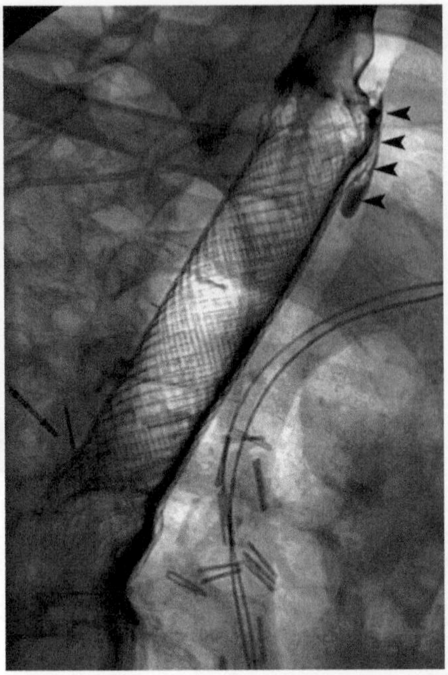

Fig. 4. Stent leakage ("endoleakage") around the proximal ending of an esophageal stent (*arrowheads*) between the stent body and the esophageal wall.

and should be discussed in detail with the anesthesiologist before starting the procedure. Moreover, during the intervention very honest and professional communication is essential. Without this, a fatal outcome is more likely. It is important to prepare everything before starting the procedure, including positioning of fluoroscopy, choosing the right stent, and connecting all cables, thus shortening the time under general anesthesia and the duration of the intervention itself. Tracheal stenting requires a rigid bronchoscopy and general anesthesia to relax the patient. Maintaining sufficient ventilation can be difficult, if not impossible, in a patient with a wide patent TEF. Passing the fistula with the bronchoscope, and ventilating the patient through the bronchoscope lying distally to the fistula, is usually possible without problems in a high TEF. However, in a fistula at the level of the tracheal bifurcation this is not feasible, and jet-ventilation is mandatory.

Continuous percutaneous monitoring of O_2 and CO_2 is essential in such unstable respiratory situations, and the anesthesiologist and the interventionist must be prepared to allow periods without any ventilation. After the best possible preoxygenation, the patient will tolerate several minutes without ventilation. The interventionist must be brave and experienced enough to quickly complete the stenting in an apneic phase, if necessary. Interrupting the intervention to treat hypoxia will not always help to improve oxygenation. The worst possibility is to leave the field and responsibility to an inexperienced and panicked anesthesiologist in a situation when the saturation decreases dramatically. This situation will often result in a fatal outcome as the anesthesiologist tries, without success, to intubate and ventilate the patient conventionally. This action is prone to failure as ventilation pressure is lost via the patent TEF into the esophagus.

Choosing the correct tracheal stent

In TEF, self-expandable stents have some advantages over rigid silicone stents. Self-expandable stents can be placed more easily, and be deployed over a guide wire or even under direct vision (**Fig. 5**). Malpositioning of the stent can quickly lead to a dangerous situation if the stent placement cannot be corrected or the stent is not withdrawn quickly enough. These corrections are also easier with this type of stent. The dimensions of the expanded stent should be 4 cm longer than the fistula, in the best scenario, so that the coated part overlaps for about 2 cm on each side of the TEF. Sixty millimeters is a standard length; longer may be necessary, and shorter will often prove too short afterward. The TEF may become wider and longer with time because of pressure necrosis by the stent, especially in a double-stent situation. Diameters of 20 mm fit in most tracheas, with 18 mm being sufficient for slimmer patients. It may help to measure the size of the healthy trachea on the CT scan, but if in doubt the larger size should be chosen. A firm sitting of the stent

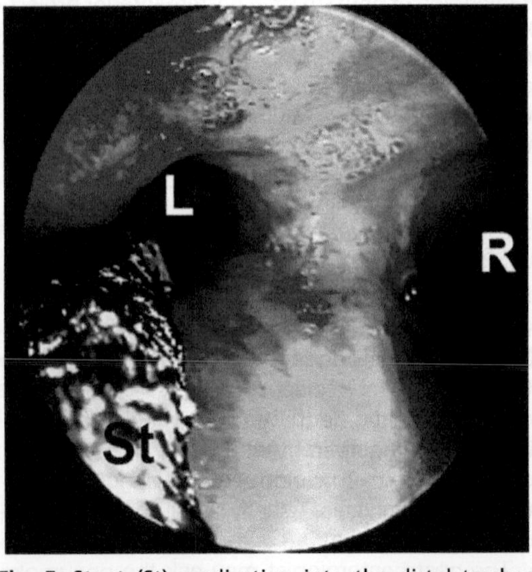

Fig. 5. Stent (St) application into the distal trachea under visual bronchoscopic control. L, left main bronchus; R, right main bronchus.

is more likely to produce granulation tissue at its ends. This problem is not a major one for these patients with a short life expectancy, and can be accepted for achieving a secure sealing of the fistula if esophageal stenting has failed. When the tracheal orifice of the fistula is close to the carina (see **Fig. 2**), a self-expandable Y-stent is advisable, again with the largest dimensions possible that fit the patient.

Stenting technique

Whereas a normal straight stent can often be deployed without fluoroscopy, it is mandatory in positioning a Y-stent. It is advisable to position the fluoroscopy unit correctly before beginning the procedure, and to mark the level of the main carina and the edges of the fistula with radiopaque marks on the patient's skin.

The authors always prepare a rigid and a flexible scope, and intubate the patient with the widest rigid tracheoscope that fits through the larynx, mostly #12 or, better, #14. The distal end of the tracheoscope is positioned in the proximal trachea and secured there by an assistant. Through this wide rigid scope the 0° rigid optic, as well as the flexible scope, can be inserted, even alongside the suction probe or the stent applicator (see **Fig. 5**).

A normal straight stent can often be quickly positioned under direct vision with its distal end well below the fistula orifice, and deployed under optical control without using a guide wire or fluoroscopy (see **Fig. 5**). When stenting under visual control only, special attention is needed to ensure the distal tip of the stent applicator is positioned in the trachea and not, via the fistula, in the esophagus! It is wise to position the stent a little too deep and then pull it back as much as needed afterward. Pushing the stent deeper after deploying it too high is very difficult and will likely lead to damage to the stent.

Endoscopic surveillance of positioning the Y-stent is impossible, owing to the diameter of the applicator. When placing a Y-stent, the 2 guide wires are introduced in both main bronchi (**Fig. 6**) through the flexible scope under optical and fluoroscopic control. The 2 bronchial arms of the Y-stent are introduced over the 2 guide wires. Utmost care must be taken that these wires do not cross inside the trachea but run parallel when introducing the stent over these wires. During the opening of the 2 bronchial stent parts, constant firm contact of the stent bifurcation to the tracheal carina must be maintained and controlled fluoroscopically. During this phase, the patient cannot be ventilated. After both bronchial arms have opened completely, the tracheal part is released.

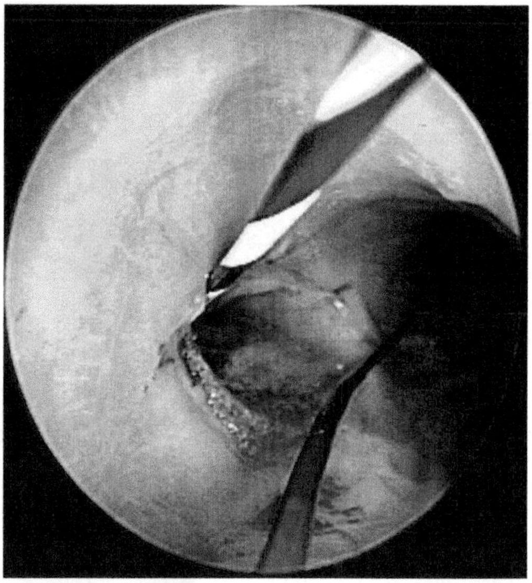

Fig. 6. Two guide wires to the left and right main bronchus, the first step of positioning a Y-stent. Typically, the 2 wires are still crossing inside the trachea and will be untwisted under fluoroscopic control by turning the Y-stent applicator in the appropriate direction while advancing it.

Immediately afterward, the stent position is endoscopically controlled. Whenever a Y-stent is malpositioned, ventilation may be impossible. Emergency extraction of the stent with the rigid scope will require relevant force, but may be the only chance to save the patient.

The "Unstentable" Fistula

Fistula into one main bronchus is very difficult to seal by tracheobronchial stenting if esophageal stenting is not successful or not possible. Frequently some leakage will persist after airway stenting, giving only partial relief to the patient. When the fistula is close to the carina (see **Fig. 2**), the authors first place a Y-stent with the longer bronchial part into the fistula-bearing bronchus and, if necessary, put another stent (**Fig. 7**) into this bronchial arm. This action may lead to overstenting the upper lobe bronchus, especially on the right side. Fortunately, fistulas develop more frequently on the left side.

Fistulas to the most peripheral bronchi or the lung parenchyma cannot be sealed by stenting. If the side of the lung to which the fistula leads is already destroyed, or at least functionally not relevant to the patient, it can be sacrificed by overstenting it with a tracheobronchial stent to the remaining healthy lung. This action may stop the episodes of aspiration and coughing, but will not stop the process of aspiration-related

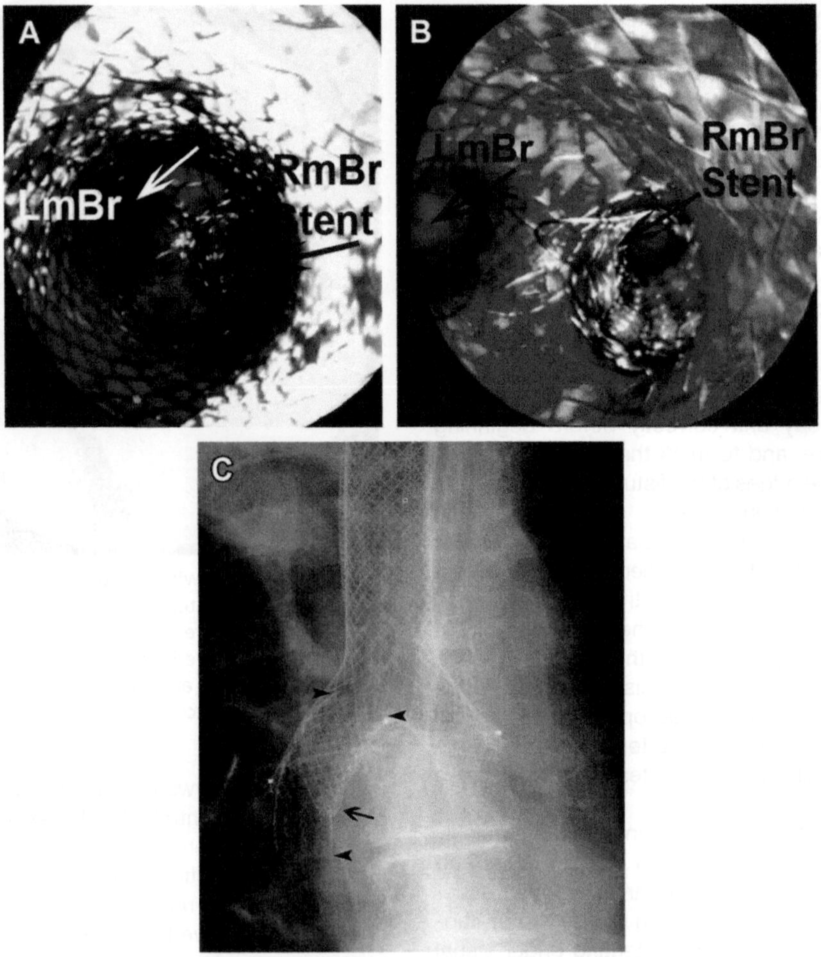

Fig. 7. (*A*) Y-Stent with "stent in stent" (RmBr Stent) into the right main bronchus. LmBr, left main bronchus. (*B*) Stent in stent: closer view of the same situation as in *A* (labeling same as in *A*). (*C*) Stent in stent: radiograph of the same case. Bronchial stent (*arrowheads*) prolonging the Y-stent's right bronchial distal end (*arrows*); the Y-stent was inserted in a reverse manner, so that the normally longer left arm is positioned in the right main bronchus. The origin of the right upper lobe bronchus was intentionally "overstented" to cover a fistula in the short right main bronchus.

infection to the now excluded lung, thus, perhaps, ending in fatal necrotizing pneumonia. Obviously this can only be a final option to alleviate symptoms for a patient close to death, and must be combined with long-term broad-spectrum antibiotics.

Interventional filling of the peripheral fistula tract with histoacryl, through a catheter under fluoroscopic guidance, is an experimental treatment. This technique can be used to seal a peripheral fistula without sacrificing too much lung function and without long-term infectious consequences. However, this is possible only in close cooperation with an experienced radiologist. The procedure resembles angiographic embolization, with the important difference that contrast medium is not washed out by the bloodstream. It accumulates as in bronchography and, with alveolar overfilling, can worsen visualization of the fistula tract and lead to pulmonary dysfunction and infectious problems in this lung area. Intermittent suction removal of the contrast medium with the flexible bronchoscope helps, but will not completely avoid this effect of endobronchial spillage.

If it remains impossible to close the fistula completely, percutaneous endoscopic gastrostomy or percutaneous endoscopic jejunostomy is unavoidable, and should always have been discussed with the patient before stent placement. Sometimes solid food can be swallowed to a limited extent, but drinking mostly remains impossible with persistent TEF. It is worth testing whether swallowing in certain body positions reduces aspiration.

Tracheostomy, and positioning a blockable cannula with its balloon distally to the fistula, can avoid aspiration in very high persistent fistula. A persistent tracheostomy with cutaneotracheal anastomosis should be created with a suction tube, wide enough to allow the cleaning of ingested substances from the trachea proximal to the balloon, without the need to remove the tracheal cannula every time. Special cannulas have inserts into an outer blockable cannula that allow the patient to speak with the blocked cannula in place. This insert can easily be exchanged with a closed version before eating or drinking, by the patient or his or her relatives, and the outer cannula remaining in place avoids misplacement.

Typical Problems After Double Stenting of Trachea and Esophagus

Whenever double stenting of the trachea and esophagus cannot be avoided, this will compress the remaining walls of the esophagus and the trachea between the 2 stents and may induce tissue necrosis, thus further increasing the original fistula size. Another important consequence of double stenting in the narrow upper mediastinum is that a secondarily placed esophageal stent may not open adequately (see **Fig. 3**B, C), despite correct size and even after additional balloon dilatation. This situation should not be falsely attributed to tumor stenosis, and repeated dilatation will not help. Esophageal stents have widening ends to help secure the position of the stent. If this widening part lies at the level of the tracheal stent, it may not have enough space to expand fully to the outside. Instead it will invert into the lumen of the esophagus, thus obstructing it. Pulling back the esophageal stent to a position where its proximal orifice lies orally to the tracheal stent will help (see **Fig. 3**D, E), but is only possible if the fistula is not too high and if the chosen esophageal stent is not too short.

POSTINTERVENTIONAL MANAGEMENT AND HOME CARE

Esophageal stents pose fewer problems and maintenance issues in comparison with tracheal stents. The patient should be advised to chew food very well and to swallow sparkling liquid with the food to avoid stent obstruction. Many of these patients lack their natural teeth, and their prosthesis often sits too loose after progressive weight loss and mandibular atrophy. Food should be pureed before offering it to a patient unable to chew properly.

Tracheal stents require frequent humid inhalations, preferably every hour during daytime, to avoid incrustation of secretions in the stent (**Fig. 8**). If there is suspicion of clotting in the stent, bronchoscopy should not be postponed, because these secretions can become so hard that they cannot be removed without damaging the stent coating. Moreover, they can lead to total obstruction of the stent.

RESULTS OF TEF STENTING

Complications and Mortality

Taking into account the often frail condition of the patients, and the demanding peri-interventional airway management in TEF, peri-interventional and procedure-related mortality is reported as surprisingly low: from 0% to 2%.[5] It has been reported as higher, at 14.6%[11]; however, in this study, of 4 deaths only 1 was directly attributable to the stenting procedure because of esophageal perforation, leading to a 2.4% stenting-related mortality. The other deaths were more related to unsuccessful stenting and disease progression.

Complication and mortality rates are often reported for a whole group of stenting patients, as in the series of Sarper and colleagues,[11] and not for the small subgroup of stenting in TEF. Groups who publish large case studies tend to have appropriate experience, and it may be speculated that fatal outcome is more to be feared in less experienced hands but often will not be published. In fact, data in the literature on mortality in stenting for TEF are scarce, and no data are available on the frequency and outcome of these procedures outside experienced centers.

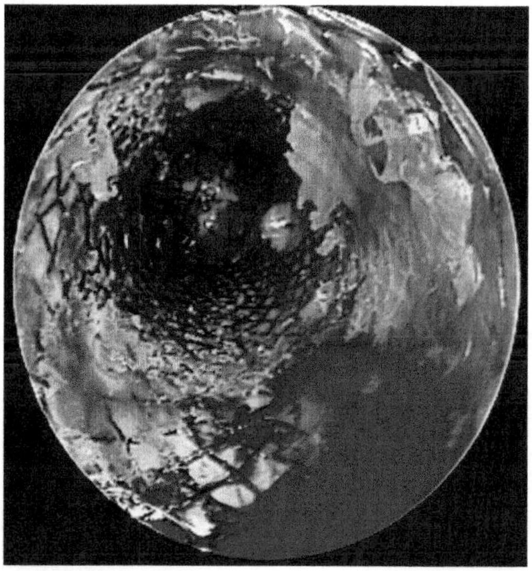

Fig. 8. Incrustations inside a tracheobronchial Y-stent that may soon lead to complete obstruction.

One secondary complication after successful stent placement can be stent migration, typically of the esophageal stent, after single stenting. In double stenting, the mutual pressure of the stents mostly avoids stent migration but can cause enlargement of the fistula, and thus the reopening of the TEF. Adding or replacing a stent can sometimes manage reactivation of the mTEF.

One problem of covered stents is the fragile nature of the covering material, especially if the stent has been cleaned mechanically to treat stent obstruction, as the covering can suffer small perforations that are not easily recognized during endoscopy of a sedated patient. However, the higher abdominal pressure in the awake patient, and the gastroesophageal reflux that is frequently observed in these patients, can induce significant aspiration episodes through these small holes. The authors have lost one patient as a result of massive acute aspiration from a huge mediastinal necrosis cavity through the wall of a tracheal Y-stent.

Bronchial stents need to be sized as large as possible, which provokes formation of granulation tissue at the stent's margins (**Fig. 9**). The lumen of the smaller distal bronchial orifices of a Y-stent (see **Fig. 9**) or tracheobronchial single-lumen stent can be obstructed by granulation tissue and scarring. Again, treating these granulations bronchoscopically with forceps, laser, or in the authors' hands preferably with an argon beamer, must be done with greatest care so as not to damage the stent coating.

Survival After TEF Stenting

The study of Chen and colleagues[4] demonstrated that early closure of the fistula improved survival in their patients compared with mere feeding gastrostomy or jejunostomy, probably by avoiding early deaths caused by aspiration pneumonia, whereas long-term survival is dominated by the underlying oncologic disease. These data confirmed the results of a larger study of 264 patients from Balazs and colleagues,[5] which showed a 3-fold increase in mean survival in patients with successful stenting from 1.1 months to 3.4 months. Remarkably, in the surgical series of Davydov and colleagues[1] a rather high mortality of 14.3% was the price for a much better median (13 months; range 3–31 months) and 2-year survival (21%) in this select group. Perhaps esophageal surgeons and their oncologic partners should rethink palliative treatment and local control of advanced disease by considering multivisceral resection as a primary treatment option whenever it seems feasible, and before mTEF can develop and the patient is still in good condition. A life expectancy at the time of initial diagnosis of 10 months in these patients[5] could justify aggressive surgery, thus to avoid TEF as a devastating complication of the disease.

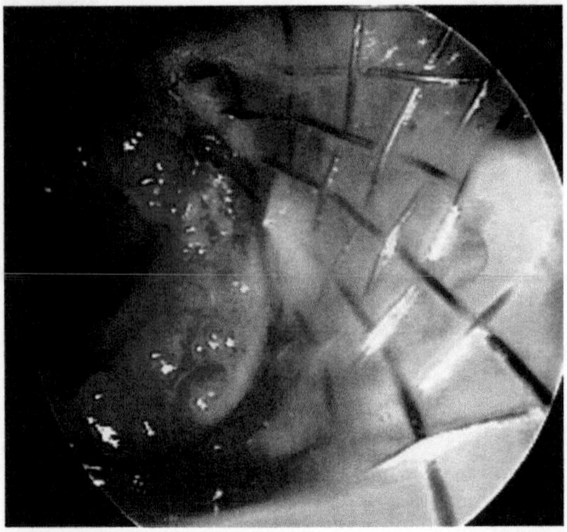

Fig. 9. Granulations at the distal bronchial ending of a Y-stent.

REFERENCES

1. Davydov M, Stilidi I, Bokhyan V, et al. Surgical treatment of esophageal carcinoma complicated by fistulas. Eur J Cardiothorac Surg 2001;20(2): 405–8.
2. Reed MF, Mathisen DJ. Tracheoesophageal fistula. Chest Surg Clin N Am 2003;13(2):271–89.
3. Shin JH, Song HY, Ko GY, et al. Esophagorespiratory fistula: long-term results of palliative treatment with covered expandable metallic stents in 61 patients. Radiology 2004;232(1):252–9.
4. Chen YH, Li SH, Chiu YC, et al. Comparative study of esophageal stent and feeding gastrostomy/jejunostomy for tracheoesophageal fistula caused by esophageal squamous cell carcinoma. PLoS One 2012;7(8):e42766.
5. Balazs A, Kupcsulik PK, Galambos Z. Esophagorespiratory fistulas of tumorous origin. Non-operative management of 264 cases in a 20-year period. Eur J Cardiothorac Surg 2008;34(5):1103–7.
6. Kim KR, Shin JH, Song HY, et al. Palliative treatment of malignant esophagopulmonary fistulas with covered expandable metallic stents. AJR Am J Roentgenol 2009;193(4):W278–82.
7. Miyata T, Watanabe M, Nagai Y, et al. Successful esophageal bypass surgery in a patient with a large tracheoesophageal fistula following endotracheal stenting and chemoradiotherapy for advanced esophageal cancer: case report. Esophagus 2013; 10(1):27–9.

8. Saxon RR, Barton RE, Katon RM, et al. Treatment of malignant esophagorespiratory fistulas with silicone-covered metallic Z stents. J Vasc Interv Radiol 1995; 6:237–42.
9. Wang MQ, Sze DY, Wang ZP, et al. Delayed complications after esophageal stent placement for treatment of malignant esophageal obstructions and esophagorespiratory fistulas. J Vasc Interv Radiol 2001;12:465–74.
10. Devière J, Quarre JP, Love J, et al. Self-expandable stent and injection of tissue adhesive for malignant bronchoesophageal fistula. Gastrointest Endosc 1994;40:508–10.
11. Sarper A, Oz N, Cihangir C, et al. The efficacy of self-expanding metal stents for palliation of malignant esophageal strictures and fistulas. Eur J Cardiothorac Surg 2003;23(5):794–8.

Index

Note: Page numbers of article titles are in **boldface** type.

A

Acute postoperative respiratory compromise
  and tracheal resection, 20
Adenoid cystic carcinoma
  tracheal, 73–76
  and tracheal tumors, 9
  treatment in advanced tracheal cases, 75, 76
Air conditioning
  by the trachea, 3, 4
Airway collapse
  and tracheomalacia, 52–56
Airway management
  and carinal resection and sleeve pneumonectomy, 21, 22
  and tracheobronchial injuries, 41–46
  and tracheobronchial surgery, 18
  and tracheobronchomalacia, 23
Airway stenoses
  and tracheobronchial surgery anesthesia, 17
Airway transplantation, **97–106**
  and immunosuppressive medication, 98–102, 104
  and tissue rejection, 98, 99, 101
  types of, 97, 98
Allogenic cells
  vs. autologous cells in tracheal tissue engineering, 102
Anastomosis
  and cricotracheal resection, 69, 70
  dehiscence of, 114, 115
  and sleeve pneumonectomy, 21, 22
  and tracheal surgery complications, 111, 114, 115
Anesthesia
  for carinal resection and sleeve pneumonectomy, 78
  for laryngotracheal resection, 67, 68
  for tracheal resection, 67, 68
  during tracheobronchial surgery, 16–23
Anesthesia and gas exchange in tracheal surgery, **13–25**
AO. See *Apneic oxygenation.*
Aortopexy
  and tracheomalacia, 57
Apneic oxygenation
  clinical aspects of, 15
  and hypercapnia, 15
  and pulmonary arterial carbon dioxide, 15
  and pulmonary oxygen, 15
  and respiratory acidosis, 15
  and tracheobronchial surgery, 15
Apneic reflex
  of the trachea, 4
Aspirated microorganisms
  removal of, 4
Autologous cells
  vs. allogenic cells in tracheal tissue engineering, 102

B

Barotrauma
  and jet ventilation, 14
Benign stenosis of the trachea, **59–65**
Benign tracheal stenoses, 31–39, 59–64
  after tracheotomy, 59, 60
  and bronchoscopy, 61
  causes of, 59–61
  and clinical signs, 61
  and computed tomography, 61, 62
  cuff-induced, 60, 61
  diagnosis of, 61, 62
  and extension into the larynx, 63
  and idiopathic inflammation, 61
  and indications for treatment, 62
  and lung function testing, 61
  and operative access, 62
  pathomechanisms of, 59–61
  and postoperative care, 63
  and resection with anastomosis, 62, 63
  and results of treatment, 64
  symptoms of, 61, 62
  treatment of, 62–64
Benign tracheal strictures
  stents in, 35–39
  treatment of, 31–33
Benign tracheal tumors
  treatment of, 31
Bioreactor
  and tracheal tissue engineering, 102, 103
Bleeding
  and tracheal surgery complications, 111, 112
Botali ligament
  division of, 88
Breathing
  and tracheal reflexes, 4
Bronchoscopy
  and benign tracheal stenoses, 61
  and tracheal surgery complications, 109

Thorac Surg Clin 24 (2014) 129–134
http://dx.doi.org/10.1016/S1547-4127(13)00160-6

C

Cadaveric aorta
  and tracheal allotransplantation, 99
Cadaveric tracheas
  in allotransplantation, 98, 99
Cardiopulmonary bypass
  and tracheobronchial surgery, 16
Carinal resection
  without pulmonary resection, 80
Carinal resection and sleeve pneumonectomy, **77–83**
  and airway management, 21, 22
  and anastomosis, 21, 22
  anesthesia for, 78
  and anesthetic complications, 22, 23
  contraindications for, 78
  and extensive resections, 80
  and gas exchange, 21, 22
  history of, 77, 78
  indications for, 78
  and left sleeve pneumonectomy, 80
  and lung cancer, 78
  and morbidity and mortality, 81, 82
  patient selection for, 78
  and postoperative care, 80, 81
  and right sleeve pneumonectomy, 79, 80
  surgical technique for, 79, 80
  and ventilation techniques, 21, 22
CEA. See *Cervical extradural anesthesia.*
Cervical extradural anesthesia
  in extrathoracic tracheal surgery, 16
  physiologic effects of, 16
CFI-V. See *Cross-field intubation-ventilation.*
Chemotherapy
  for tracheal cancer, 76
Children
  tracheomalacia in, 52, 57
Chronic obstructive pulmonary disease
  and surgery for tracheomalacia, 56
Combined modality treatment
  for tracheal cancer, 75
Computed tomography
  and benign tracheal stenoses, 61, 62
  and tracheomalacia, 53, 54
Conduct of anesthesia
  and tracheobronchial surgery, 17
  and tracheobronchomalacia, 23
Cough reflex
  of the trachea, 4
CPB. See *Cardiopulmonary bypass.*
CR. See *Carinal resection.*
Cricotracheal resection
  and anastomotic technique, 69, 70
  surgical technique for, 69, 70
Cross-field intubation-ventilation
  and tracheal resection, 18–22
Cryorecanalization
  and tracheal stenoses, 29, 30
Cuffs
  and benign tracheal stenoses, 60, 61

D

Dilatation
  and tracheal stenoses, 34, 35

E

ECMO. See *Extracorporeal membrane oxygenation.*
Embryonic development
  of the trachea, 3
Emphysema
  and tracheobronchial injuries, 42, 43, 46
Endoscopic treatment of tracheal stenosis, **27–40**
Endoscopy
  and tracheal stenoses, 27–39
  and tracheomalacia, 54
Endotracheal tubes
  and high-frequency jet ventilation, 19
Epithelial precursor lesions
  and tracheal tumors, 8, 9
ETT. See *Endotracheal tubes.*
Expiration reflex
  of the trachea, 4
Exsiccation
  and jet ventilation, 14
Extended tracheal resections, **85–95**
  and carinal resection and sleeve pneumonectomy, 80
  and division of botali ligament, 88
  and intrapericardial hilar release, 88
  and mobilization of pretracheal plane, 87, 88
  and pericardiophrenic release, 88
  and pneumoperitoneum, 90
  and reimplantation of left main bronchus, 88–90
  and results of treatment, 90–93
  and suprahyoid laryngeal release, 88
  and suprathyroid laryngeal release, 88
  and tracheal reconstruction, 86, 90, 91
  and tracheal-release techniques, 87
Extracorporeal gas exchange
  during tracheobronchial surgery, 16
Extracorporeal membrane oxygenation
  and tracheobronchial surgery, 16
Extrinsic compression
  and tracheomalacia, 55

F

Fiberoptic bronchoscopy
  and tracheobronchial surgery anesthesia, 13, 16–18, 20–23
FOB. See *Fiberoptic bronchoscopy.*

G

Gas exchange
and carinal resection and sleeve pneumonectomy, 21, 22
and tracheobronchial surgery, 13–16
and tracheobronchomalacia, 23
Granulomas
and tracheal surgery complications, 114

H

HFJV. See *High-frequency jet ventilation.*
High-frequency jet ventilation
and alternatives in tracheal resection, 18
and endotracheal tubes, 19
and laryngeal mask airway, 18, 19
limitations of, 20
and respiratory physiology, 14
and sequence of techniques, 19
settings for, 19, 20
technical considerations for, 18
and tracheal resection, 18–20
and tracheostomy cannula, 19
Hypercapnia
and apneic oxygenation, 15
Hypothermia
and jet ventilation, 14

I

Iatrogenic tracheal membrane lacerations, 46–49
Idiopathic inflammation
and benign tracheal stenoses, 61
IGRT. See *Image-guided radiotherapy.*
Image-guided radiotherapy
and tracheal cancer, 74, 75
Immunosuppressive medication
and airway transplantation, 98–102, 104
IMRT. See *Intensity-modulated radiotherapy.*
Inhalational anesthesia
and tracheobronchial surgery, 17
Inspired debris
removal of, 4
Intensity-modulated radiotherapy
and tracheal cancer, 74, 75
Intrapericardial hilar release
and extended tracheal resections, 88
Intubation
and surgery for tracheomalacia, 55, 56

J

Jet ventilation
and barotrauma, 14
and exsiccation, 14
and gas pressures, 14
and gas volumes, 14
and hypothermia, 14
and tracheobronchial surgery, 13–15
JV. See *Jet ventilation.*

L

Laryngeal mask airway
and high-frequency jet ventilation, 18, 19
Laryngotracheal resection
anesthesia for, 67, 68
complications of, 71
and incision and exposure, 68
indications for, 67
and postoperative care, 70, 71
surgical technique for, 68–70
Laryngotracheal resection and reconstruction, **67–71**
Larynx
and benign tracheal stenoses, 63
Laser resection
and tracheal stenoses, 28–34, 37
Left main bronchus
reimplantation of, 88–90
LFJV. See *Low-frequency jet ventilation.*
LMA. See *Laryngeal mask airway.*
Low-frequency jet ventilation
and tracheobronchial surgery, 14
Lung cancer
and carinal resection and sleeve pneumonectomy, 78
Lung function testing
and benign tracheal stenoses, 61

M

Malignant salivary gland–type tumors
of the trachea, 9, 10
Malignant tracheal stenoses
and extrinsic tumor compression, 31
nonobstructing, 30, 31
obstructing, 28–30
treatment of, 27–31
and wall destruction, 31
Malignant tracheoesophageal fistulas
and complications of stenting, 125, 126
diagnosis of, 118
epidemiology of, 117, 118
and esophageal stenting, 119–121
and postintervention care, 125
and results of stenting, 125, 126
and stenting of trachea and esophagus, 125
and survival after stenting, 126
symptoms of, 118
and tracheobronchoscopic stenting, 121–123
treatment of, 117–126
and unstentable fistulas, 123–125
Management of tracheal surgery complications, **107–116**

Mestastasis
and tracheal tumors, 8, 9
mTEF. See *Malignant tracheoesophageal fistulas.*
Mucosal inflammation
and tracheal surgery complications, 110
Multipotent stem cells
in tracheal tissue engineering, 101, 102

N

Noniatrogenic tracheobronchial injuries, 41–46

O

Operative access
and benign tracheal stenoses, 62
for tracheobronchial injuries, 45

P

Pain therapy
and tracheobronchial surgery anesthesia, 17
Pathology of tracheal tumors, **7–11**
Penetrating tracheobronchial injuries, 44, 45
Pericardiophrenic release
and extended tracheal resections, 88
Pharmaceutical intervention
and tracheal tissue engineering, 103, 104
Photodynamic therapy
and tracheal stenoses, 30
Pluripotent stem cells
in tracheal tissue engineering, 101
Pneumoperitoneum
and extended tracheal resections, 90
Pretracheal plane
mobilization of, 87, 88
Pulmonary arterial carbon dioxide
and apneic oxygenation, 15
Pulmonary oxygen
and apneic oxygenation, 15
Pumpless interventional lung assist
and tracheobronchial surgery, 16

R

Radiological findings
and tracheal surgery complications, 109
Radiotherapy
for tracheal cancer, 74–76
Repair of tracheobronchial injuries, **41–50**
Respiratory acidosis
and apneic oxygenation, 15
Restenosis
and tracheal surgery complications, 115
RT. See *Radiotherapy.*

S

Scaffolds
in tracheal tissue engineering, 100, 101
Secondary tumors
of the trachea, 9
Sleeve pneumonectomy
and carinal resection, 21–23, 77–82
left, 80
right, 79, 80
SP. See *Sleeve pneumonectomy.*
Spasmodic reflex
of the trachea, 4
Squamous cell carcinoma
and surgical results, 74
tracheal, 73–76
and tracheal tumors, 9
Stem cells
of the trachea, 2, 3
in tracheal tissue engineering, 101, 102
Stents
and benign tracheal strictures, 35–39
and malignant tracheoesophageal fistulas, 125, 126
Stoma
and surgery for tracheomalacia, 55, 56
Strictures
and tracheal stenoses, 31–39
Suprahyoid laryngeal release
and extended tracheal resections, 88
Suprathyroid laryngeal release
and extended tracheal resections, 88
Systemic palliative chemotherapy
for tracheal cancer, 76

T

TBI. See *Tracheobronchial injuries.*
TBS. See *Tracheobronchial surgery.*
TE. See *Tissue engineering.*
Terminally differentiated cells
in tracheal tissue engineering, 102
Tissue engineering
and tracheal reconstruction, 99–104
Tissue rejection
and airway transplantation, 98, 99, 101
TML. See *Tracheal membrane lacerations.*
TNM classification
of tracheal tumors, 8
Total intravenous anesthesia
and tracheobronchial surgery, 17
Trachea
and air conditioning, 3, 4
air transport in, 3
anatomy of, 1
and apneic reflex, 4
and cough reflex, 4
embryonic development of, 3
and expiration reflex, 4
functions of, 1–4
histologic findings, 2

morphogenesis of, 1, 2
physiology of, 3
and rapid shallow breathing, 4
and removal of aspirated microorganisms, 4
and removal of inspired debris, 4
and slowing of breathing, 4
and spasmodic reflex, 4
and stem cells, 2, 3
and tube diameter, 4
Trachea: anatomy and physiology, **1–5**
Tracheal allotransplantation
and cadaveric aorta, 99
chemically preserved, 99
cryopreserved, 99
fresh cadaveric, 98, 99
irradiated, 99
in situ processed fresh cadaveric, 99
Tracheal cancer
and adenoid cystic carcinoma, 73–76
combined modality treatment for, 75
and image-guided radiotherapy, 74, 75
and intensity-modulated radiotherapy, 74, 75
radiotherapy for, 74–76
and squamous cell carcinoma, 73–76
surgery for, 73, 74
and systemic palliative chemotherapy, 76
treatment of, 73–76
and volumetric intensity-modulated arc therapy, 74, 75
Tracheal membrane lacerations
classification of, 46
diagnosis of, 46
iatrogenic, 46–49
surgery for, 47
symptoms of, 46
treatment of, 46, 47
Tracheal release
and extended resections, 85–88
Tracheal replacement, 97–104
and tissue engineering, 99–104
Tracheal resection
and acute postoperative respiratory compromise, 20
with anastomosis, 62, 63
anesthesia for, 67, 68
complications of, 71
and cross-field intubation-ventilation, 18–22
and emergence from anesthesia, 20
extended, 85–94
and high-frequency jet ventilation, 18–20
indications for, 18, 67
and postoperative care, 20, 70, 71
and reconstruction, 70
surgical technique for, 68, 69
and termination of surgery, 20
Tracheal stenoses
benign, 31–39, 59–64
and cryorecanalization, 29, 30
and dilatation, 34, 35
endoscopic treatment of, 27–39
and laser resection, 28–34, 37
malignant, 27–31
and photodynamic therapy, 30
and strictures, 31–39
and tracheal surgery complications, 111
Tracheal surgery complications
and anastomotic site, 114
and anesthesia, 22, 23
and bleeding, 111, 112
and bronchoscopy by surgeon, 109
and dehiscence of anastomosis, 114, 115
and granuloma formation, 114
and intraoperative measures, 110
and laryngotracheal resection, 71
and level of stenosis, 111
and mucosal inflammation, 110
operative management of, 112–114
and patient history, 109
and planning of operative procedure, 108, 109
postoperative, 111–115
and postoperative care, 110
prevalence of, 107, 108
prevention of, 108–110
and radiological findings, 109
and resection of wrong trachea level, 111
and restenosis, 115
and stenting, 125, 126
and tension of anastomosis, 111
during tracheal resection, 110, 111
and tracheo-innominate artery fistula, 111, 112
and tracheobronchial infection, 110
and ventilation, 110, 111
Tracheal tissue engineering
and artificial scaffolds, 100, 101
and autologous vs. allogenic cells, 102
and biologic scaffolds, 100
and bioreactor, 102, 103
cells for, 101, 102
and composite scaffolds, 101
and multipotent stem cells, 101, 102
and pharmaceutical intervention, 103, 104
and pluripotent stem cells, 101
scaffold-free, 101
and scaffolds, 100, 101
and stem cells, 101, 102
and terminally differentiated cells, 102
Tracheal tumors
and adenoid cystic carcinoma, 9
epidemiology of, 7
and epithelial precursor lesions, 8, 9
malignant salivary gland–type, 9, 10
and mestastasis, 8, 9
pathology of, 7–10
and premalignant lesions, 8, 9

Tracheal (*continued*)
prognosis of, 10
secondary, 9
and squamous cell carcinoma, 9
TNM classification of, 8
World Health Organization classification of, 7, 8
Tracheo-innominate artery fistulas
and tracheal surgery complications, 111, 112
Tracheobronchial infections
and tracheal surgery complications, 110
Tracheobronchial injuries
and airway management, 41–46
diagnosis of, 42, 43
and emphysema, 42, 43, 46
management of, 43
mechanisms of, 42
and membrane lacerations, 46–49
noniatrogenic, 41–46
operative access for, 45
penetrating, 44, 45
repair of, 41–49
statistics for, 41, 42
surgery for, 43, 44
Tracheobronchial surgery
anesthesia during, 16–23
and apneic oxygenation, 15
in awake patients, 15, 16
and cardiopulmonary bypass, 16
and cervical extradural anesthesia, 15, 16
extracorporeal gas exchange during, 16
and extracorporeal membrane oxygenation, 16
gas exchange during, 13–16
and jet ventilation, 13–15
and low-frequency jet ventilation, 14
and pumpless interventional lung assist, 16
and sleeve pneumonectomy and carinal resection, 21–23
and tracheal resection, 18–20
and tracheobronchomalacia, 23
Tracheobronchial surgery anesthesia
and airway management, 18
and airway stenosis, 17
conduct of, 17
and diagnostics, 16, 17
equipment for, 17, 18
and fiberoptic bronchoscopy, 13, 16–18, 20–23
inhalational, 17
monitoring of, 17, 18
and pain therapy, 17
total intravenous, 17
Tracheobronchomalacia
and airway management, 23
and conduct of anesthesia, 23
and gas exchange, 23
Tracheobronchoscopic stenting
and anesthesiologic peri-interventional management, 121, 122
and choosing the correct stent, 122, 123
technique for, 123
Tracheoesophageal fistulas
malignant, 117–126
Tracheomalacia, **51–58**
and airway collapse, 52–56
and aortopexy, 57
in children, 52, 57
classification of, 51, 52
and computed tomography, 53, 54
diagnosis of, 52–54
endoscopic treatment for, 54
and extrinsic compression, 55
and surgery after intubation, 55, 56
and surgery after stoma, 55, 56
surgery for, 54–57
and surgery in chronic obstructive pulmonary disease, 56
therapy for, 54, 55
Tracheoplasty
and tracheomalacia, 56
Tracheostomy cannula
and high-frequency jet ventilation, 19
Tracheotomy
and benign tracheal stenoses, 59, 60
Treatment approaches to primary tracheal cancer, **73–76**
Treatment of malignant tracheoesophageal fistula, **117–127**
Tube diameter
of the trachea, 4
Tumor compression
and malignant tracheal stenoses, 31

V

Ventilation
and tracheal surgery complications, 110, 111
VMAT. See *Volumetric intensity-modulated arc therapy.*
Volumetric intensity-modulated arc therapy
and tracheal cancer, 74, 75

W

Wall destruction
and malignant tracheal stenoses, 31
Web stenoses
treatment of, 33
World Health Organization classification
of tracheal tumors, 7, 8

Printed and bound by CPI Group (UK) Ltd, Croydon, CR0 4YY
03/10/2024
01040370-0004